Radiant Wellness

A Holistic Guide for Optimal Earthly Experiences

Mark Pitstick, MA, DC

All inquiries should be addressed to:
Mark R. Pitstick, MA, DC
center@radiant101.com
7407752189

Radiant Wellness:
A Holistic Guide for Optimal Earthly Experiences
by Mark Pitstick, MA, DC $19.95 ISBN 978-0-9661419-9-3

(Previously published as Balanced Living: Transforming Body, Mind, and Spirit)

Warning/Disclaimer

Every effort has been made to make this collection of materials as complete and accurate as possible. Nevertheless, information may change, and there may be mistakes, both typographical and in content. Important data may be omitted. Therefore, this book should be used as a general guide only and not as the only source of information.

Further, all statements made by the author are based on his own personal research and study; they do not necessarily reflect the beliefs of all professionals. In no way is any information contained herein meant to take the place of or to provide any kind of professional advice or treatment. Nor does it preclude the need to seek the advice of professionals on a personal level.

Acknowledgements

To my beloved family and friends

To my teachers and patients who have taught me so much

To Dr. Paul Brown, Otto and Susie Collins, Lainey Ebright, Brooke King, Andy Lee, Lucy Lather, Rae Lynn Pitstick and Virginia Pitstick for their editorial assistance

To Ryan Roghaar for the interior and cover design work

To Erica Milligan for back cover photography

To the many researchers, authors, and health care practitioners from whom I have learned so much

To my Higher Energy Assistants/Assistance, thank you for all of your love, support and guidance.

To Life Source / All That Is / E.L.G.O.D., whose wondrous nature has become more obvious as I've fine-tuned my body and mind.

Table of Contents

Radiant Wellness

A Holistic Guide for Optimal Earthly Experiences

Mark Pitstick, MA, DC

Introduction

The quality of your earthly experience is directly affected by how much you really know the following and live accordingly. Much clinical and scientific evidence strongly indicates that you:

- are an eternal being of consciousness.
- do not 'lose' loved ones who pass on, but reunite with them when you change worlds.
- can enjoy a continued although different relationship with those who have dropped their physical body.
- encounter not just one, but many life experiences throughout eternity.
- are one with the One and an integral part of Life Source
- are interconnected with other people, animals, nature and all of life.
- receive assistance and guidance from sources described as angels, guides, master teachers, higher energies, and the Light.
- create how heavenly or hellish your life feels – whether on earth or elsewhere – by your predominant thoughts, words, and deeds.

Optimal self-care is one of the natural responses to knowing who you really are. And, conversely, having a balanced and vitally healthy body and mind can help you better know your true nature.

You can enjoy total success and be healthy, happy, prosperous, and peaceful. You can enjoy loving relationships, engage in meaningful lifework, and have a rock-solid spiritual foundation. That's your birthright, the way it's supposed to work. But, as the saying goes, "God helps those who help themselves." Are you willing to do your part?

I've worked with many thousands of people in hospitals, mental health centers, and holistic health centers. My books, newsletters, audio products, workshops, and multimedia interviews have helped many people around the world. Now you can benefit from my forty-five years of training and experience in medical, theological, psychological, and chiropractic fields.

As eternal beings having a very temporary human experience, you have two distinct natures. The first has been termed the *transcendent source of consciousness* (TSC), an awareness that preexists human birth and survives physical death.

As the fetus develops, a second type of awareness forms, the *brain based consciousness* (BBC). This is the awareness associated with the physical brain's activity. The BBC is affected by the wellness, or lack thereof, of your body and brain.

The quality of your life is determined by the degree to which the TSC and the BBC are *entrained or working in harmony.*

Self responsibility is a major theme in this process. For example, cigarette smoking and obesity cause nearly one million U.S. deaths per year. These are largely preventable by stopping tobacco use, eating properly and exercising.

While working in hospitals, I assisted a very obese patient who had just undergone her 12th surgery for ankle, knee and hip problems. While talking with her, I discovered she ate way too much of the wrong foods and never exercised. Hoping to plant some seeds of awareness, I remarked about the number of surgeries she had received.

"Yes," she replied, "I guess God just didn't put me together very well."

The seven keys to optimal living are relatively simple but *the power of the basics,* done on a regular basis, create outstanding results:

1. ***Renewal:*** *rest, sleep, vacation, and leisure time*
2. ***Activity:*** *exercise and fully engaging in life*
3. ***Diet:*** *the real food way of eating and whole food supplements*
4. ***Inner Cleanse:*** *healthy eliminative, detox and lifestyle practices*
5. ***Awareness:*** *attention to emotional and mental needs*
6. ***Natural Care:*** *non-drug and non-surgical health approaches to restore and maintain your health*
7. ***Transcendence:*** *realizing you're an eternal being in a totally supportive universe*

By the way, the first letter of each key spells RADIANT. That's what you really are: a radiant being of energy/spirit/awareness who is just temporarily visiting this planet for loving service, adventure, growth and enjoyment.

Again, remember that small improvements performed consistently over time can result in huge benefits. After incorporating new changes into your lifestyle, you'll soon be ready for additional improvements. Stay balanced and don't get obsessive about any one area. Do your very best and know that's good enough.

Everyone is unique so please balance my recommendations with what makes sense to you. You have an amazing innate intelligence so use it. What makes you consistently feel, look and be your very best? I'm presenting this information as *a way* that has helped many, not *the only way.*

By the way, reaching your personal best is not just a self-serving pursuit. Vibrantly healthy and well-balanced people have the greatest ability to serve others and make a real impact. Imagine the net effect on our world as more and more of us reach our fullest potential and share our greatest gifts.

Be sure to *actively read* by taking notes and highlighting pertinent sections. This book is not light reading so take a break if you start feeling overwhelmed.

Each chapter ends with a *Bottom Line* section that highlights key points. An *Action Steps* section follows so you can write down changes you plan to implement. Remember, knowledge isn't power—*knowledge combined with inspired action* is.

I recommend that you make at least two changes per month for each of the seven keys. Do this for three months and you'll enjoy over forty improvements! Notice the positive results in every aspect of your life after only ninety days! This *positive upward spiral* will motivate you to continue fine-tuning your self care program.

Here we go. You are at an important crossroads in your life right now. I hope you *play full out* and enthusiastically learn and implement this information.

Are you ready?

Renewal
A
D
I
A
N
T

Key #1
Renewal

Resting, recharging and relaxing are integral parts of holistic health. Sufficient *renewal* is a big key to feeling great and being healthy.

An old Irish proverb stated, 'The beginning of health is sleep.' As usual, it's a question of balance since sleep requirements vary widely. For example, Thomas Edison required only four hours per night while Albert Einstein preferred ten or more. Most people need about eight hours. Identify how much sleep you need to feel your best and regularly get that amount.

How do you determine how much sleep is ideal for you? Consider how many hours you need before you awaken without an alarm clock. Also, what is the amount of sleep that allows you to feel energetic throughout the day? If you can't always obtain that many hours, do so as often as possible.

The amount of sleep you need to feel great can change. Some people may need less as they get older. You may find that you require less sleep when you regularly meditate, exercise, eat healthfully, get your body balanced, and follow your passions in all areas of life.

Rest is one of the most underestimated and powerful healing tools at your disposal. Extra sleep and downtime allow the body to make adaptations and work internal miracles. Early physicians often prescribed complete bed rest because it helped so many maladies.

Listen to your inner wisdom and take time for extra renewal when you just don't feel right. Lighten your schedule, go to bed earlier, cancel social engagements, and get a nap. Extra rest can mean the difference between just feeling under the weather for a day versus getting a fullblown illness.

When faced with significant physical or emotional challenges, the body conserves its energy for healing and survival. It's natural to feel tired when you are excessively stressed or fighting off an illness. Your body is telling you to rest and lay low for awhile. I sometimes hear patients complain that they have been tired lately, but "are too busy to slow down."

They ignore these messages and keep pushing themselves, perhaps with the aid of stimulants like nicotine, sugar or excess caffeine. Then a severe cold or flu—with unpleasant symptoms and lost work time—*makes* them take a break.

Rest, vacation, leisure, play, and "creative laziness" are important aspects of life. Learn to say "no" to the constant requests and demands on your time. Carve out quality time for you and your family; everyone will be happier and healthier for it. Regularly enjoy hobbies and leisure activities. If possible, transition to a four-day work week. Take a three-day weekend periodically.

Use your full allotment of vacation days and, when you do take a vacation, really enjoy it. Leave the extra work and laptop computer at home. You'll be more healthy, efficient and happy by taking time for rejuvenation.

Healthy Sleep Habits

- ***Open your bedroom window,*** *just a crack during cold weather, to ensure adequate oxygen and fresh air while sleeping. This is especially important if your heating and cooling system recirculates inside air instead of drawing in fresh air.*

- ***Be asleep by 10:30 pm,*** *even earlier when needing extra rest. Midnight was so named because it was the middle of the night for our ancestors. The saying "early to bed, early to rise, makes a person healthy, wealthy, and wise" is good counsel.*

  Natural health experts say the hours of sleep before midnight are the most beneficial. Staying up late is also counterproductive because it often results in excessive TV viewing, computer or video game use, and late night eating.

- ***If necessary, take a daily nap*** *that confers many benefits for relatively little time required. Just a 1530 minute nap provides deep rest and releases accumulated stress.*

Optimal Sleep Strategies

Sleeping deeply throughout the night is a major key to radiant wellness. Natural approaches to help you do this include:

1. ***Avoid eating a heavy dinner****—especially later in the evening—so you don't experience indigestion that interrupts sleep. However, if hunger pangs keep you awake, have a light healthy snack before bedtime.*
2. ***Minimize your caffeine intake*** *(coffee or tea) to only one or two servings per day with none after mid-afternoon to avoid excess stimulation. Avoid soda pop of any type and sugary snacks because of the over stimulation and for many other reasons.*
3. ***Quit smoking*** *since nicotine is a potent stimulant of the nervous system and disrupts sleep with coughing.*
4. ***Go to bed and arise at about the same time*** *each day so your body gets on schedule.*
5. ***Use your bedroom*** *only for sleeping and amorous activities.*
6. ***Obtain corrective chiropractic care*** *to ensure optimal alignment of your spine, especially the neck. If vertebrae are out of alignment, sleep positions can worsen nerve pressure and make it difficult to sleep soundly.*
7. ***Keep your bedroom*** *dark, quiet, and cool.*

8. ***If you suffer with insomnia,*** *avoid naps since that might throw off your sleep schedule. Stay awake through the day so you'll be tired and better able to sleep at night.*

9. ***If your brain races*** *when you try to sleep, touch forehead relaxation points for five minutes while thinking of any worries. Rest your middle three finger pads on the frontal protuberances, those bumps a few inches above your eyebrows. Breathe slowly and deeply and process your worries.*

10. ***Regularly exercise,*** *but not in the evening.*

11. ***Relieve stress*** *of the adrenal glands, brain, cardiovascular system and thyroid. Each of these organs, when imbalanced, can cause insomnia. A holistically trained physician can recommend a natural program to balance these.*

12. ***Consider whole food nutritional supplements*** *to help calm the body and mind.*

13. ***Get a great medical and natural health care checkup*** *to rule out any significant problems that may be causing insomnia. Consider natural remedies such as hypnosis therapy or acupuncture that may help.*

14. ***Use relaxation techniques*** *such as massage, hot baths, relaxation audios, soothing music or nature sounds.*

15. ***Regular meditation*** *creates a relaxed state of mind and promotes deep sleep.*

16. ***Try light therapy*** *with bulbs that emphasize the blue color spectrum if your insomnia is worse during months with less sunlight,*

17. ***Pray and intend*** *to become aware of how you can sleep well.*

Proper Sleep Postures, Pillows and Mattresses

You spend about one-third of your life in bed so proper sleep postures, a good pillow and mattress are very important.

1. ***Sleep on your back and side.*** *Avoid stomach sleeping because it twists the neck and can exert pressure on nerves and blood vessels.*

2. ***Periodically change positions*** *throughout the night to prevent excessive pressure on the hips and shoulders.*
3. ***Use only one medium thickness pillow*** *so the neck is not bent. The memory foam brands seem to hold their shape and are comfortable.*
4. ***A firm conventional mattress*** *with a pillow top surface is best for most people.*

Regarding waterbeds, some natural health experts question the wisdom of sleeping on water since it can absorb energy. Did our ancestors sleep on a raft while sleeping? Bottom line? Everyone is different. Find the best sleeping surface for you given your physical condition and preferences.

Slumbering Creativity

You can benefit from *creative insights* that occur just before sleep or while dreaming. Keep a notepad and pen on your bedside table to capture ideas and inspiring thoughts. Review your goals and read or listen to motivational material just before going to sleep. This fills your heart and mind with positive themes instead of absorbing the latest tragedies from the 11 o'clock news.

Parents, read quality books to your children at bedtime to feed them lofty ideals and aid language development. Just after they've fallen asleep, tell them how special, talented, and beloved they are. They will soak up those great truths and program their lives accordingly.

Finally, metaphysical wisdom holds that the soul can access other dimensions during sleep. Just because your body needs rest doesn't mean your transcendent source of consciousness must stay dormant all night. The mind processes information and conflicts during sleep. Thus, you may want more sleep when actively working on spiritual, mental or emotional issues.

Relaxation Techniques

The following strategies assist recharging and rejuvenation:

- ***Meditation and yoga*** *as discussed in the Awareness chapter*
- ***Daily stretching and exercise*** *as discussed in the Activity chapter. Brief stretching and just 20 minutes of brisk walking significantly reduces anxiety and renews your energy.*
- ***Hot baths*** *are another effective way to deeply relax. Soak the neck and upper back where tension often accumulates. Allow yourself the luxury of soaking for at least 30 minutes, especially in a hot tub or Jacuzzi spa.*
- ***Pace yourself*** *as you run the race of life. Long term studies show that calmer Type B personalities are just as or even more productive than their faster paced Type A counterparts. Life is a marathon race, not a sprint, so "easy does it".*
- ***Enjoy the ride*** *as you journey through life. My patients who live healthfully into their eighties and nineties are usually easy going and don't get too worked up about events in life.*
- ***Take time for yourself,*** *at least a little each day. You deserve some fun and relaxation every day. You'll be more productive and prosperous when you take time to play and enjoy life.*

Renewal—it's as simple as that! Optimal sleep, relaxation, vacationing, and leisure on a regular basis. Now that you know the first key to *radiant wellness,* it's time to map out your plan for improvements in this area. Remember, knowledge plus inspired action creates results so please complete the action steps.

———◆———

The Bottom Line

The most important points in the *Renewal* chapter include:

1. *Get a deep night's sleep on a regular basis*
2. *Obtain extra rest at the first sign of illness or feeling down*
3. *Use the "optimal sleep strategies" if you have trouble getting or staying asleep*
4. *Meditate for deep physiological rest and other benefits*
5. *Consider a daily nap if your health status, sleep patterns, stress or activity levels require it*
6. *Enjoy regular vacations, long weekends, and lazy days*
7. *Spend time doing enjoyable hobbies and leisure activities*

Action Steps for Renewing Your Life

List two action steps you commit to starting within 30 days:

1. ______________________________
2. ______________________________

List two action steps you commit to starting within 60 days:

1. ______________________________
2. ______________________________

List two action steps you commit to starting within 90 days:

1. ______________________________
2. ______________________________

R
Activity
D
I
A
N
T

Key #2
Activity

Regularly enjoying the *right amount and type of activity* is another key to reaching total vibrancy of body, mind, and spirit.

One of my mentors, Jack LaLanne, DC, is a remarkable example of how we can look, feel, and function throughout our lives. On his 70th birthday, he swam one mile while pulling 70 small boats containing friends and local residents.

Years later, after showing film footage of his latest feat, a TV host gushed, 'Jack, you're amazing—I don't know how you do it!' Jack quickly interjected, 'You're missing the whole point! I'm not amazing. This is how we all can be if we take care of ourselves and use more of our potential!' He went full-speed until age 96 and demonstrated what is possible. To see for yourself, visit his website at ***JackLaLanne.com***.

Benefits of Exercise

Exercise is a prime example of how you can positively alter your life with relatively little time and effort. Proper exercise need not be time consuming, difficult, or expensive. The many benefits of exercise include:

- *Strengthening and flexibility of muscles, tendons and ligaments*
- *Looking your best with good muscle tone and posture*

- *Weight loss due to burning calories during exercise and at an accelerated rate for 12 to 24 hours afterward*
- *Production of brain chemicals that create a postexercise euphoria (the runner's high) that makes you feel great naturally*
- *Suppressed and more easily controlled appetite*
- *Deeper and longer sleep patterns*
- *Increased self-esteem and personal mastery*
- *Bone strengthening and prevention or reversal of osteoporosis*
- *Conditioning of the nervous system and reflexes*
- *A zenlike reverie during exercise*

Are these sufficient reasons for you to exercise and stretch for just a few hours a week?

Maintaining lean muscle mass helps you look, feel, and act better at any age. Young people have much more muscle than fat; this contributes to their increased energy, higher metabolism, greater strength and balance, and more active lifestyle. Without regular exercise and proper diet, older people develop more fat than muscle. That starts a downward spiral of fatigue, weight gain, weakness, poor balance and restricted lifestyle.

The phrase *make your life a work of art* has always been motivating to me. Have pride in your physique just as you do in your car and home. It's healthy to feel proud of yourself when you look your best. Post pictures of how you want to look and use them as motivation to create the body you deserve.

The human body is a magnificent creation and a wondrous thing to behold when we are lean and fit. Unfortunately, many people today have a pear-shaped body due to lack of exercise and improper diet. Just look around—70 percent of Americans are overweight and over 1/3 are obese. How they feel and function suffer accordingly.

If you're overweight, guidelines for reaching your ideal weight include:

1. *Keep active with regular exercise and an energetic lifestyle*
2. *Eat moderate amounts of real food and take whole food supplements as discussed in the Diet chapter*
3. *Use nutritional healing methods as discussed in the Natural Care chapter*

Guidelines for Exercise

If you haven't exercised for a while, take it slow and easy at first. Trying to exercise too much too soon is a common reason that exercise programs fail. After overdoing it, you'll feel sore, tired, and unwilling to suffer again. Build yourself into shape steadily using graduated steps. Kenneth Cooper, M.D., considers aerobic exercise very safe for all ages if six basic guidelines are followed:

1. ***Get a physical examination*** *within a year of starting an exercise program, within 3 months if you're over 40.*
2. ***Watch your diet and control weight,*** *blood sugar and cholesterol levels. Wait at least 2 hours after a heavy meal before exercising vigorously.*
3. ***Warm up*** *with stretches and slow walking.*
4. ***Don't overexert;*** *stop exercising if you experience chest pain, severe shortness of breath, dizziness, or nausea.*
5. ***Cool down*** *by tapering off exercising during the last five minutes to prevent nausea, cramps, and soft tissue strains.*
6. ***Avoid gaps in your program.*** *Stick with your exercise schedule, especially during the first ten weeks of a new program.*
7. ***The three components of exercise*** *are aerobic conditioning, resistance training, and stretching. Let's examine each one in more detail.*

Aerobic Conditioning

Traditional recommendations have been to exercise steadily and intensely enough to maintain your heart rate at (220 your age) x 70% for 45 minutes, four days a week. This approach has been widely accepted over time and provides good results.

Recent research supports *interval training* as described by Phil Campbell in *Ready, Set, Go!* and Al Sears, M.D., in *Pace: Discover Your Native Fitness.* Interval training involves short intervals of full speed exertion mixed with more moderately paced breaks for recovery. It requires only twenty-minute workouts, three times a week. Typically, a thirty-second full out period occurs every two minutes. Benefits are increased calorie burning and greater aerobic training in less time.

Consult a fitness instructor about the best program for you given your goals and health status.

Cardiovascular benefits can be achieved with any the following approaches IF your target heart rate is reached and maintained as described above:

- *Brisk walking outdoors or using a treadmill*
- *Jogging: same as above*
- *Ski machines like the NordicTrack or cross country skiing*
- *Aerobic dance*
- *Workout machines such as the stair stepper and elliptical units*
- *Biking: stationary, spinning, or on the road*
- *Rowing via a machine or in the water*
- *Racquet sports if you keep active between points and games*
- *Sustained integrated exercise programs such as Pilates and Ashtanga Yoga*

Cross training involves using two or more types of exercise each week for a more complete workout and change of pace. Listening to music or audio programs while exercising indoors helps alleviate boredom. For safety reasons, I don't recommend this while exercising outdoors.

Resistance Training

Resistance or strength training can be done with weights, therabands, ashtanga yoga, Pilates, or traditional floor exercises. Consult a certified exercise instructor who can design and oversee the best program for you. Two to three sessions a week of 45 to 60 minutes each are sufficient for most fitness goals.

Functional fitness involves exercise that mirrors everyday activities. Muscle groups are developed in a more integrated way using balance, low weight, stabilizer balls and other devices. In the beginning, a person's body weight is sufficient to obtain benefits. Later, small dumbbells are added. Functional exercises train muscles to work together while increasing core muscle strength, balance, flexibility and agility.

Recommended books on this topic are *Functional Training* by Juan Carlos Santana, M.Ed., CSCS, and *Core Performance* by Mark Verstegen and Pete Williams. Dr. Sears recommends a more naturally oriented approach to fitness that prepares a person for activities of daily living. Excellent DVD programs include those by Tracy Anderson, Mandy Ingber, Rodney Yee, Elisabeth Halfpapp and Fred DeVito, and others.

For more traditional weightlifting approaches, I recommend two programs. The first involves using machines with very slow movements and relatively low weight. *The Slow Burn Fitness Revolution* by Fredrick Hahn, Mary Eades, M.D., and Michael Eades, M.D., thoroughly describes this approach. *Body for Life* by Bill Phillips discusses a weight training approach using dumbbells and machines. Using dumbbells versus machines enhances neuromuscular development by involving other muscle groups to maintain proper form.

Here's a simple key to performing resistance exercises more easily and powerfully. Just remember E-E which means *exhale during exertion.* For example, with bench presses, take a deep breath, exhale while slowly pushing the weight above your chest, and then inhale again as you lower the weight to your chest. Use this same breathing pattern during any strengthening exercise.

The following *floor exercises* strengthen core muscles. If your fitness level allows, do these on an exercise ball for greater benefits. If you're out of shape, start with just a few repetitions and increase slowly over time.

- ***Sit-ups*** *should be performed with the knees bent and by just raising the shoulder blades off the floor. Hold that position or do crunches with repetitive abdominal flexion. Imagine that you are squeezing water out of a sponge as you focus on contracting your abdominal muscles.*

  For the abdominal obliques or "love handles" on the side, rotate your torso to either side and hold or crunch.

- ***Pushups:*** *do slowly and with good form for maximum results*

- ***Back Extensors*** *are performed while lying face down. With your arms outstretched, raise the head, arms, chest, and legs—leaving only the pelvis on the floor. Hold for several seconds and repeat. This strengthens back muscles and aids posture and spinal stability.*

  If this is too difficult, put your hands on the floor and push just your upper body off the floor. These were called 'girl's pushups' years ago and are called the cobra pose in yoga. For the lower half, raise one leg up at a time and hold for several seconds.

- ***Leg Raises*** *strengthen lower abdominal muscles and complement sit-ups. Lie on your back with arms along your sides. Raise your legs, head and shoulders up and hold, then lower slowly.*

- ***Ball Bounces*** *involve bouncing on a ball while doing Kegel exercises to strengthen core muscles. Sit on an exercise ball so that your knees are bent at right angles and your widely spaced feet are on the floor. Bounce up and down while intermittently tightening your pelvic floor muscles as if you were holding in a bowel movement. Do for five minutes, three times a week for two weeks.*

Increase the time bouncing by five minutes every two weeks to a maximum of fifteen minutes. This simple and easy exercise efficiently strengthens muscles that stabilize the spine and pelvis. You can do these while talking, watching TV, or listening to music or informational audio programs.

Stretching

Stretching is the third component of exercise and is a natural activity when you're in touch with your body. Observe dogs or cats after a long nap: their first movements are long deep stretches, arching the back and then stretching each leg. Stretching promotes soft tissue flexibility, prevents or slows arthritic progression, and helps maintain normal skeletal and spinal alignment.

Follow these guidelines when stretching:

- *Do in the morning and more often as needed*
- *Perform slowly and avoid bouncing or jerking movements*
- *Stretch to the point of slight pulling or tightness; stop if you experience any pain*
- *If pain or limited range of motion persist, consult a chiropractor, physical therapist, or other specialist trained in biomechanics*

The following stretching program quickly covers the entire body:

- ***The Tree stretch*** *can be done standing or lying on your back. It counteracts gravitational forces by gently tractioning the spine. With arms and hands high above your head, stretch until you feel a slight pull along the back*
- ***Neck range of motion stretches*** *involve moving your head forward, backward, looking over each shoulder, and side bending with your ear toward each shoulder.*
- ***Trunk twists*** *stretch the thoracic spine or mid-back. While standing with your feet at shoulder width apart, keep immobile below the waist while twisting the upper torso back and forth to each side. Keeping your arms outstretched facilitates full range of motion.*

- ***Side bends*** *stretch the lumbar spine, sacroiliac joints, and hip sockets. While standing, bend to the side and run your fingertips along the outside of the thigh toward the knee.*
- ***Back bends*** *help maintain the normal lateral low back curve and alignment of lumbar vertebrae. While standing, place your hands over the tailbone or in the small of your back and stretch backwards.*
- ***Hamstring stretches*** *benefit muscles on the back of the thigh. Lie on your back and raise one leg up while keeping the knee joint straight. Grab behind the knee with both hands to assist stretching of these muscles.*
- ***Calf stretches,*** *the "runner's stretch," work the hamstrings and calf muscles. Hold onto something for stability while standing with one foot outstretched behind you. Keep up on your toes and ball of that foot as you stretch the heel toward the ground.*
- ***Quadriceps stretches*** *aid the muscles on the front of the thigh. While standing, stabilize yourself with one hand and grab your ankle with the other hand. Pull your heel toward your buttocks and feel the quadriceps stretch.*
- ***Groin stretches*** *are for the inner thigh and groin muscles. Sit with both feet near the crotch and let your knees stretch down toward the floor.*
- ***Knee chest pulls*** *stretch low back muscles and are done while lying on your back. Pull first one, then the other, then both knees to the chest as far as possible.*
- ***Shoulder stretches:*** *with arms outstretched, do circular rolls one way and then the other. Next, move your arms forward and backward, then above your head and down to the sides.*

Integrated Techniques

Several integrated techniques provide numerous benefits: stretching, strengthening, skeletal alignment, deep breathing, enhanced awareness, internal organ massage and proper posture.

Yoga is the oldest system that provides these benefits; excellent programs are now widely available. For many years, I used the *Integral Hatha Yoga* program taught by Swami Satchidananda. In *Fountain of Youth,* Peter Kelder describes ancient rites or postures purportedly used by Tibetan Lamas to aid longevity and vital functioning in all areas of life. I use these basic movements each morning as a warm-up. Ashtanga yoga provides many body/mind/spirit benefits and is an excellent integrated approach.

The Pilates Method is another integrated approach to strengthening muscles while improving balance and flexibility. Components of this approach include mental concentration, precise and flowing movements, specific positions and focused breathing.

Moshe Feldenkrais pioneered body movement and awareness work with his "Functional Integration" technique. W. Reich, F.M. Alexander, Ida Rolf, Fritz Perls, and Alexander Lowen were other early teachers of integrated techniques. Specific stretches can reprogram healthy neuromuscular patterns while de-programming aberrant ones.

Fully Engaging in Life

Being dynamic is the final step for optimal activity. Observe how lean people move quickly, keep busy, and have lots of energy for projects. They like to be active, even if it's helping with the dishes or picking up the house.

An old adage states: "To become, act as if." So model the behavior of people who are trim and slim. How can you become a more active person? You know the basics: exercise regularly, park farther away, climb stairs instead of using elevators, put on your sneakers and pick up the pace while cleaning the house, and do your own yard work.

Exercising on a regular basis allows you to fully participate in life's activities without paying for it afterward. When you're fit, you can enjoy diverse recreation, play with your children or grandchildren and pets, and spend time in nature. These activities are part of a rich and varied life.

Design your life to include more activities. For example, enjoy time with family and friends while walking in nature, biking, kayaking or canoeing. Take dance, yoga, or martial arts lessons with your loved ones for an active evening out. Ice skating, roller skating, bowling, ping pong and billiards are other fun activities. Enjoy a family swim and participate in team sports. Be creative and come up with your own ways to add more activity to your life.

Activity—it's as simple as that!

Don't like to exercise? An interviewer of Jack LaLanne mentioned that he must be one of those rare individuals who *enjoys* exercising. Jack responded, 'I work out every day *and I hate it.* But, I love the way I feel. I love the way my body works and I love the way I look. So I do it." His comments helped me because, like most people, I have to push myself to get started. But I'm always glad I worked out and feel better afterwards.

Optimal activity requires only a few hours per week of stretching, cardiovascular conditioning, and strengthening. In addition, maintain an active lifestyle and make more robust lifestyle choices. Then you can enjoy the game of life and increasingly experience radiant wellness!

———◆———

The Bottom Line

The most important points in the Activity chapter include:

1. *Aerobic exercise at least three times per week for 2030 minutes*
2. *Resistance training two to three times per week*
3. *Stretch each morning and more often if needed*
4. *Use integrative techniques like yoga that combine numbers 1 to 3*
5. *Develop the habit of being active and fully engaged in life*
6. *Enjoy exercise and other activities with family and friends*

Action Steps for Optimal Activity in Your Life

List two action steps you commit to starting within 30 days:

1. ________________________________
2. ________________________________

List two action steps you commit to starting within 60 days:

1. ________________________________
2. ________________________________

List two action steps you commit to starting within 90 days:

1. ________________________________
2. ________________________________

RADIANT Diet

Key #3
Diet

Even though you are an eternal being of energy/spirit, your physical body has certain requirements. How you eat can make your time on earth seem like heaven or hell for you and others around you. What's more, your way of eating can make a huge difference in how you treat yourself and others.

Remember, it's very difficult to know who you really are and live accordingly when you are suffering with fatigue, anxiety, depression, brain fog, chronic pain, etc. And your way of eating plays a major role in these and many other symptoms.

Here's an example. Ed was a fourteen-year-old boy who suffered with bloody diarrhea ten to twelve times a day and was diagnosed with Crohn's disease. Ed couldn't sleep at night because of the diarrhea and often had to run out of his classroom at school to use the bathroom. His greatest fear was having uncontrollable diarrhea in front of his classmates.

I can guarantee you he wasn't feeling very radiant.

Ed's condition worsened despite six years of treatment with medical drugs. A permanent colostomy—removing his colon and installing a bag for his intestinal wastes—was discussed. His medical doctors never recommended any dietary changes or other natural approaches to assist digestion and calm inflammation. Just drugs, then surgery. Inexcusable.

Fortunately, someone told his parents about holistic health care. I'll share how his story ended at the close of this chapter.

Much research clearly indicates that the following are major causes of disease and early death: sugars, processed foods, and refined grains. Other causes of disease include *excess* dairy products, meat, alcohol, and caffeine, *and any tobacco.*

This is not new information. In 1941, Surgeon General Dr. Thomas Parran noted that many Americans are physically inferior and mentally dull because of their chronically poor diet.

Are you going to *eat to live or live to eat?* Food *tastes* good for only a few seconds before swallowing. After that, it improves or impairs your health. Wouldn't you rather eat more healthfully and feel great than eat unhealthfully and feel miserable?

Don't worry, you don't have to completely avoid offending foods. Most people can *occasionally* have junk foods IF they eat healthfully most of the time.

Here's a suggestion: go to a grocery where unhealthy foods are sold. Observe the person pushing the grocery cart, then look at what they are buying. If the person looks and moves like a zombie, their cart will likely include lots of pop, white bread, pastries, canned, and other poor quality "foods."

In a short time, you can increasingly enjoy the taste of fresh real foods. Try this challenge: eat healthfully – the real food way of eating – for just thirty days and then revisit your old fast food restaurants, conventional grocery stores, and vending machines.

If you're like most people, processed junk foods will now taste sickeningly sweet and artificial. What's more, you'll feel fatigue, brain fog, and depression soon afterwards. In the next day or two, your joints and muscles will feel sore and stiff while your gastrointestinal system complains loudly.

Optimal nutrition is really very simple:

1. *Drink lots of pure water.*
2. *Enjoy the real food way of eating with moderate amounts of healthy, chemical-free, nonGMO foods.*
3. *Take whole food supplements as needed.*

Until very recently on an evolutionary scale, there were no refined, artificial, or heavily sugared foods. Hunters and gatherers primarily ate vegetables, fruit, nuts, seeds, lean meats, and eggs. The only available sweet was honey and that required outfoxing an entire bee hive. Their beverage of choice? Pure water.

Archeologists say that these ancient ancestors were much healthier than we are. They were tall, lean, and robust. They had much less degenerative disease, arthritis, tooth decay, cancer, and heart disease than modern day humans. How? They ate healthfully, were active, took time to enjoy hobbies and interactions with others, drank pure water, and enjoyed moderate sunshine. Simple, right?

Now, fast forward to the 21st century...

People of all ages, including children, are developing all manner of physical and mental symptoms because of nutritional deficiencies. They are often deluged with chemicals, heavy metals, and microorganisms that abound in food, air, water, vaccinations, medical drugs, body care products. In addition, their bodies are assaulted by a tsunami of electromagnetic fields from all the electronic devices, cell towers, etc.

And people wonder why there's such an increase in depression, anxiety, alcohol and drug abuse, addiction, illness, memory loss, violence, suicide, and murder?

You may not realize the seriousness of the situation because most people don't talk about their embarrassing symptoms. However, every holistic physician knows how many people suffer with an alarmingly large list of physical and mental problems. Top integrative medical doctors like Mark Hyman MD recognize how many people suffer with 'broken brains.'

I recently spoke about holistic health care at a retirement village. Afterwards, an older couple came up to thank me. He was 92 and still jogged everyday; she was 89 and taught yoga. Hailing from Germany, they both stood straight and were lean, bright eyed, mentally sharp, and took no medical drugs. They shared how shocked they were when they came to the U.S. and saw how many people took numerous prescription drugs. In Europe, they said, people spent more money on healthy food, activities, and enjoying a healthier and more interesting life.

You can be the same way with some consistent changes in your self-care habits. Let's dive in... what can you do to improve your health and that of your loved ones?

First, you must educate yourself. As discussed in Michael Pollan's books *The Omnivore's Dilemma* and *In Defense of Food,* the terms "organic" and "free-range" have been misused by the food industry. Organic is usually a trustworthy term but be careful. For example, the term 'organic eggs' may only mean that chickens are given healthy feed, but are still raised in cramped cages throughout their lives. "Free range" eggs can merely mean that hens had access to a small concrete pen during half of their short lives.

That's why it's wise to spend extra time, energy and money to find healthy food sources for you and your loved ones. The words you can currently trust are *pasture-raised, chemical-free, nonGMO, and organic* (most of the time.) Some use the term "beyond organic" for locally-raised, sustainable agriculture sourced products. These are available at farmer's markets, small-scale local farms, and healthier grocery stores.

Pasture-raised means the animals spend significant time in grassy fields. The farmers use land and crop rotation practices that benefit the soil and the animals. In these settings, fowl eat insects and grubs in addition to chemical-free grains. Cattle primarily eat a variety of meadowland grasses, not cheap corn that produces fat marbling.

Fish should be *wild-caught,* not pond-raised since the latter are fed chemicals, antibiotics, and artificial foods.

Watch the movies *Food, Inc., Knives Over Forks, Fast Food Nation and Fat, Sick and Nearly Dead* to realize the problems created by poor diet and some solutions.

Until recently, *all food was organic* because no pesticides, herbicides, growth hormones or antibiotics were used to raise crops and animals. Now you have to pay extra for healthy food, but it's worth the increased taste, nutrients, and purity. As more people buy organic foods, prices will decrease and availability will increase.

Think you can't afford real food? Do the math. You will save several thousands of dollars each year by avoiding soda pop, tobacco, junk food, convenience foods, recreational drugs, and excess alcohol. You will save money by eating smaller portions of nutrient dense food since you reach satiety more quickly. Finally, when you're taking great care of yourself, you'll eventually most likely need fewer or no prescription medications—an additional savings.

You will then be able to afford chemical-free food, whole food supplements, a health club membership, a water filtration system, and natural health care.

I've made numerous dietary refinements over the years until I found the combination that works best for me. Ultimately, *how you feel and function* are the best barometers for what you should eat. Use the principles in this book as guidelines. Work with your health care team until you have found the right formula for you.

Before changing the way you eat, you should consult your health care providers, especially if you are on any medication or have a diagnosed illness. Whole foods exert powerful effects and your doctors should know what dietary and supplement changes you are making.

For example, after eating more healthfully and losing weight, people may need fewer or no drugs to lower blood sugar, blood pressure and cholesterol. Those taking blood thinners may need their medication adjusted when eating more foods or supplements with vitamin K.

Let's examine the various components of a healthy way of eating in more detail...

Water

How much water should you drink? One formula for ounces per day is your body weight divided by two or three. For example, if you weigh 180 pounds, you should drink 60 to 90 ounces of water a day. You may need even more if you are very active and sweat a lot. Listen to your body and follow the thirst signals.

Use certified bottled or filtered water purified by multiple stage filtration to remove impurities and improve taste. Reverse osmosis and steam distillation are great ways to purify water but remove some minerals so be sure to take whole food mineral supplements.

Most flimsy plastic water bottles are filled with boiling water. This can cause microscopic plastic particles to leach into the water. These molecules can *mimic hormones* and act as endocrine disruptors that alter the function of the thyroid gland and other organs. Read *Detoxify or Die* by Sherry Rogers MD for more information.

Use stainless steel metal water bottles (without any paint because it chips) or heavy plastic bottles (recycling symbol #2, 4 or 5 with polyethylene or polypropylene plastic). Fill these with filtered water for optimal health and to eliminate the mountain of flimsy plastic water bottles wasted each day.

What is the only liquid that falls out of the sky and replenishes its supply? That is a big hint about what you're supposed to drink.

Sadly, the average American now drinks more soda pop than water. Those who continue this habit over time will suffer physically, mentally and emotionally. This is especially true for children who begin drinking soda pop at an early age. Fortunately, schools are increasingly providing healthier alternatives.

Healthy Fats and Oils

Healthy fats are vital for health; that's why certain ones are called *essential fatty acids.* Omega-3 oils are usually needed in larger amounts in the average diet. These are found most abundantly in cold water fish: *wild-caught* salmon, mackerel, herring, tuna, and sardines. Cold processed fish oils from pristine sources, flaxseed oil, and flaxseeds are other ways to obtain sufficient omega-3 essential fatty acids.

Omega-6 and omega-9 oils are found in vegetable oils too abundant in the *Standard American Diet* (SAD). They are also in meat and eggs. The ratio of omega-3 to omega-6 oils should be 1 to 1. For the average American, this ratio is 1 to 20, thus the importance of supplementing omega-3 oils and limiting processed foods containing or cooked in vegetable oils.

Minimize or avoid saturated fats with "trans" or hydrogenated fats found primarily in fatty meats, margarine, fried foods, and processed crackers, breads, and pastries. These have been linked with increased heart disease, stroke, cancer, hypertension, diabetes, obesity, and other degenerative diseases.

Butter, especially from pasture-raised animals in the spring, is a good fat when used in moderation. *Mono-unsaturated fats,* an important part of a balanced way of eating, are found in olives and olive oil, avocados, and raw nuts. The fat in egg yolks is mostly the "mono" variety. Cook with olive oil, sesame seed oil, coconut oil, grapeseed oil, or ghee (clarified butter).

Many health experts agree that eggs from pasture-raised chickens are a great food that provide quality protein and other essential nutrients. Eggs contain lecithin that helps the body utilize the cholesterol unless you have a rare predisposition to high cholesterol called familial hypercholesterolemia.

I've eaten four eggs per day, three times per week for decades and my cholesterol levels are normal. When using the real food way of eating, many patients eat eggs and see their cholesterol levels *decrease.*

Note: Many medical and natural physicians consider the new norms for total cholesterol (below 200 mg/dL or even lower) to be driven by pharmaceutical company based or influenced studies. These numbers set the stage for many adults "needing" expensive and dangerous cholesterol-lowering medication with severe potential side effects such as liver and heart damage. People over seventy years old may actually need *more* cholesterol.

A similar problem exists with blood pressure. Good medical studies indicate a better norm for people over 60 who do not have kidney disease or diabetes is 150/90. Despite this, many seniors are still given potentially dangerous blood pressure medication to reach the supposed 120/80 norm.

For more information about these critically important topics, I recommend Julian Whitaker MD; Al Sears MD; Joseph Mercola DO; Mary Hyman MD; and Bruce West, DC.

Protein

How much protein should you eat? Depending on whom you study, recommended amounts and types of protein vary depending on your blood type, body type, oxidizer type, activity levels, and ethics. Some recommend no animal protein, whereas others on the other end of the spectrum consider it essential.

Sufficient protein is necessary for optimal body repair, lean muscle mass, optimal blood insulin levels, and essential nutrients.

One rule of thumb is that you should eat, two or three times per day, an amount of protein that is the size and thickness of the palm of your hand. This system allows for more or less protein based on your body size. For meat, that's 4 to 6 ounces per serving; for eggs, 2 to 4 a day.

Another guideline is that your protein intake in grams per day should roughly equal your body weight divided by three or four. Body builders and serious athletes may require higher levels.

For more information the optimal amounts and types of protein, read *The Protein Power Life Plan* by Michael Eades MD and Mary Eades MD, and *The Schwarzbein Principle: The Program* by Diane Schwarzbein MD. They explain how eating the right kinds and amounts of proteins, fats, and carbohydrates can help normalize metabolism, cholesterol levels, blood pressure, blood sugar levels, weight, and numerous mental and physical symptoms.

Meat, eggs, and dairy contain the most significant levels of protein. *As mentioned, only pasture-raised* animal products or wild caught fish are recommended since other sources often contain growth hormones, antibiotics, and other chemicals. Many of these substances are known to cause or are suspected of causing cancer, birth defects, or other health problems. Non-pastured animal sources also involve mistreatment of animals and result in unhealthy products. Neither is conscionable.

The Eades' book contains charts with recommended grams of protein per meal depending on your gender, height, and weight.

How much protein is in different foods? Approximate amounts are shown below:

- *Meat (fish, poultry, beef): 7 grams per ounce of meat*
- *Eggs: 6 grams per whole egg; 4 grams for egg white only*
- *Hard cheeses (mozzarella, provolone, goat): 7 grams per ounce*
- *Curd cheeses (cottage, feta, ricotta): 7 grams per ¼ cup*
- *Protein powders (plant-based, rice or whey): 2030 grams per serving*

Unless you're allergic to soy, small amounts of fermented soy products—tempeh, miso, and natto—are OK. Tofu, although not fermented, may be eaten in small amounts by most people and contains 5 grams of protein per ounce.

However, a growing number of doctors agree that *other soy products* (protein isolates, protein powders, textured protein, milk, cheese, ice cream) may contain harmful chemicals such as phytic acid and estrogen precursors and therefore are not recommended. Soy has become one of the most common allergy producing foods and offers few, if any, health benefits.

Animal products contain the most significant levels of protein. However, for different reasons, some people do not want to eat flesh foods. There are several good options for those who do not want to contribute to animals being killed. I already discussed eggs under *Fats*. Raw nuts and seeds and their butters contain some protein as do plants. Small amounts of fermented and organically raised soy products are another source of protein.

Plant-based and whey protein powders, bars, and drinks are another source of quality protein with only 5 grams of carbs per serving. Avoid brands with refined sweeteners, chemicals, and high amounts of carbohydrates. Just because a product is in a "natural food" section or store doesn't mean it's healthy. *Read the labels.* Some popular and very tasty "health bars" contain 40 or more grams of carbs.

Semi-vegetarianism – eating healthy dairy, fish, and/or eggs but no animal meat – works well for many people. If you want to eat this way for health or higher consciousness reasons, read books on healthy vegetarianism by Diane Schwarzbein MD and John McDougall, MD.

The word *moderation* is one key. The average person *in the world* eats 87 pounds of meat a year. The *average American* eats over 275 pounds per year. Six ounces of meat a day, four days a week equals 77 pounds per year.

If you can tolerate dairy products, consume moderate amounts of *certified raw* cheese, milk, or yogurt from healthfully and pasture-raised cows, goats, sheep, or buffalo. Flash-pasteurized and non-homogenized organic sources are the next best choice. For sources of healthy dairy products in your area, visit ***RealMilk.com.***

Many natural health experts advise against eating dairy products – *especially from factory-raised animals* in large commercial operations – for the following reasons:

- *Is it natural? Humans are the only species that drink the milk of another animal and drink any milk past infancy. Cow's milk is designed to support the rapid growth of baby cows and people eat more dairy products than they did a hundred years ago. Is this one reason why over 20% of children and 70% of adults in the U.S. are overweight?*
- *Many people are intolerant of dairy products and suffer distressing sinus, intestinal, mental, and other symptoms one or two days after consuming them.*
- *Dairy products, especially processed varieties from unhealthfully raised animals, are one of the most common causes of allergies and other inflammatory reactions.*
- *Antibiotics, growth hormones, and chemically-laden feed are common in many commercially raised dairy products.*
- *Pasteurization kills enzymes and alters the quality of the food while homogenization damages and alters the size of milk fats.*

"Mike" suffered with severe sinus drainage, congestion, pressure and headaches. He frequently coughed up large amounts of mucous and blew his nose. His medical doctor prescribed several different drugs that caused side effects and did not solve the underlying problem. His symptoms *completely cleared up* after he quit eating dairy products.

Like Mike, many people with chronic sinus symptoms have greatly improved simply by abstaining from all dairy for 60 to 90 days. After that, some people can reintroduce moderate amounts of healthy dairy products, especially from goat milk. Others can only tolerate small amounts occasionally or not at all.

For more information about the potential dangers of commercialized sources of milk, read: *Don't Drink Your Milk* by Frank Oski MD, former chair of pediatrics at Johns Hopkins School of Medicine, and *The Untold Story of Milk* by Ron Schmid, ND.

Carbohydrates

Many people are confused about this topic because of changing recommendations about how much and what types of carbohydrates to eat. An excessive intake of "carbs" can lead to insulin resistance, high blood sugar, excess weight, inflammation, and other common problems. Excess carbs are converted into sugars that, if not used, may be stored as fat.

Approximate grams of carbs for different food groups include:

- *Meat, poultry, and fish: very low amounts*
- *Milk, butter, and cheese: ranges from zero for butter to 12 grams per cup of milk*
- *Vegetables: most are low except moderate amounts in potatoes (15 for ½ cup)*
- *Fruits: low to moderate, but high in bananas, pears, etc.*
- *Nuts and seeds: low to moderate (2 to 7 grams for 2 TB.)*
- *Legumes: moderate to high (12 to 22 grams per serving)*
- *Grains, breads, and pastas: moderate to high (12 for slice of whole grain bread, 20 for ½ cup pasta, 51 for 5 butter crackers)*
- *Desserts and snacks: very high (27 for glazed doughnut, 48 for 10 pretzels, 60 for 1/8 of a nine inch pie)*

Some people suffer physical and mental symptoms when they eat even small amounts of carbs. An increase in yeast/fungus, virus, bacteria, and parasite populations is one possible reason since those feed on sugar. Insulin and blood sugar fluctuations are other potential causes.

Drs. Michael and Mary Eades say white sugar and flour are addictive, in part, because they exert stimulating effects on the brain similar to cocaine and heroin. That's just one reason why some people crave carbs so much: the more they eat, the more they want. Neurologist Russell Blaylock MD says that artificial sweeteners also act as neuro-excitins and neurotoxins.

Note: the following conditions warrant *strict limitation* (0 to 1 serving per day) of carbohydrates during a 90 day *healing phase:* overweight; a significant illness such as autoimmune disorder; imbalance of liver, spleen or pancreas; impaired immunity; overgrowth of virus, bacteria, yeast/fungus or parasites.

Carbohydrate guidelines for *healthy individuals* include:

1. ***If your weight and health allow,*** *eat one to two servings per day of organic legumes or grains. Legumes include: adzuki, pinto, black, garbanzo, fava, soy, red kidney, and lima beans; black eyed peas, and lentils. Grains include millet, brown rice, quinoa, and amaranth. Use sprouted grain breads and cereals by Ezekiel, Food for Life, Alvarado, and similar companies.*

2. ***Minimize gluten grains*** *(wheat, oats, rye, barley, kamut, spelt, and triticale) at least if grown in the U.S. Avoid products from grains that are sprayed with chemicals. Organic standards do not allow spraying with glyphosates, but foods labeled "natural" or "all natural" can be sprayed with chemicals and be genetically modified.*

   Some of my patients and those of other physicians in the U.S. find that avoiding wheat relieves many chronic symptoms such as headaches, joint pain, diarrhea, mental confusion, and others. Studies have not clarified whether that may be due to genetic engineering, gluten, or chemical spraying especially with glyphosates. Anecdotal reports claim that wheat in other parts of the world, Europe for example, do not cause as many problems.

3. ***Eat some raw nuts and seeds*** *that contain approximately equal amounts of protein and carbohydrates.*

4. ***Mainly eat vegetables*** *with a low glycemic (sugar) index. For example, ½ cup of potatoes contains 16 grams of sugar whereas 1 cup of romaine lettuce has only 1 gram. Higher glycemic vegetables include potatoes, peas, carrots, corn, squash, sweet potatoes and yams.*

   Nature gives valuable clues about the sugar content of fruits and vegetables. Primarily eat those that are green, red, purple, or orange; some yellow; very few white. Deeply colored vegetables contain more nutrients as well. For example, red leaf lettuce is much more nutritious than whitish-green iceberg lettuce.

5. ***Enjoy low glycemic fruits*** *in moderate amounts. For example, a small banana contains 24 grams of sugar whereas a cup of blueberries has only 5 grams. Low glycemic fruits include: raspberries, strawberries, blueberries, blackberries, grapefruit, lemon and lime.*

   Moderate varieties are apricots, cantaloupe, cherries, kiwis, grapes, pear, peaches, plums, apples and oranges. High sugar fruits include bananas, watermelon, pineapple, pears, dried fruit, and fruit juices.

6. ***Avoid processed fruit juices*** *whether in bottles, cans or frozen since they contain too much fruit sugar and can stress the pancreas and liver. The nutrients in processed fruit juices are devitalized and can contain bacterial growth. To enjoy a small amount of fruit juice, make it yourself with a juicer.*

7. ***Avoid white flour*** *and processed foods made from it: breads, crackers, pasta, and pastries—especially if they also contain sugar and trans fats.*

8. ***Avoid white sugar*** *and junk foods that contain it. Many doctors call white sugar and white flour "the white menace" because they cause so many health problems.*

Recently, an overweight patient mentioned that he's tried to lose weight for months, but to no avail. When asked about his diet, he said he had been eating lots of fruit, mainly apples and bananas. As mentioned, excess sugar can get converted to fat and contribute to insulin resistance. All this leads to fat storage, not fat burning.

Caffeine

If you choose to have any caffeine, one or two servings a day won't cause problems for most people. Caffeine—found primarily in coffee, tea, and soft drinks—stimulates the nervous system and isn't advisable for people with heart rhythm disorders, insomnia, or nervousness.

Caffeine also can irritate the bladder and cause urinary urgency and frequency. I especially recommend avoiding or minimizing caffeine if you have to get up more than once a night to urinate.

Avoid decaffeinated coffee and tea. The decaffeination process can leave chemical residues that are worse than drinking caffeine. As always, natural is best. It's better to drink a cup or two of freshly brewed coffee or tea than less decaffeinated products. Better yet, enjoy a healthy herbal substitute blend containing chicory.

You may think that you can't function without your morning caffeine, but you won't need to chemically jump start your body when you regularly follow natural health principles.

Sugar

Sugar and sugary snacks are best avoided or eaten minimally as an occasional "treat," *especially* if you are overweight or suffer with cancer, diabetes, or other serious disease. Excessive sugar intake has been directly linked to numerous physical and mental ills. Sugar also supports increased populations of yeast/fungus, parasites, viruses, and bacteria.

Less sugar, anyone?

The National Research Council, U.S. Department of Agriculture, American Heart and Cancer Associations, and the U.S. Dietary Guidelines all agree: Eat less white sugar and fewer processed foods that contain sugar. Sugar is found in many products so *read labels* and choose those with little or no sugar. Look for words that indicate additional sugar content: corn syrup, unspecified natural sweeteners, glucose, dextrose, corn sweeteners, brown sugar and fructose.

The best *natural sweeteners* are small amounts of stevia, xylitol, agave, raw honey, maple syrup, barley malt and rice syrup. Fruit concentrates, usually from grape and pear juices, are used to naturally sweeten healthy cereals and pastries. These natural sweeteners contain minerals, vitamins, and enzymes and—for most people—don't cause problems when eaten occasionally and in moderation.

Many negative reports have surfaced about *synthetic artificial sweeteners.* These include brands containing saccharine, aspartame, and sucralose. What a surprise! Maybe someday we'll get the big idea: *only real foods* are designed for consumption by humans. Changing or creating foods with technology eventually causes problems, at least in some people.

As you improve your way of eating, foods containing too much sugar will taste overly sweet. Strict regimens can be overdone, however, and become monotonous. I went without any sugar for years, but it didn't seem human to never again eat a warm chocolate chip cookie or a few bits of a hot fudge sundae.

Now I enjoy a healthy sweet (see *What Do I Eat?*) once or twice per week and rarely a couple of bites of a decadent dessert. Likewise, you can allow yourself an occasional sugary sweet *if your health status allows.*

Looking back at my childhood, I suffered with mental and physical symptoms after eating too many refined sweetened products. As a youngster, I couldn't control my sweet intake, nor was there any reason to think I should. I wondered why I felt dizzy and exhausted after eating ten cookies washed down with sugary drinks. During holidays, I binged on sweets and then felt depressed and couldn't handle excess noise and crowds.

It took many years to figure out what the problem was. My sugar intake limited my mental focus and accomplishments. It also caused recurrent upper respiratory tract infections that eventually led to a tonsillectomy. Not worth it! You can benefit from my suffering and not learn the hard way. I stay away from sugar completely when I'm tired, overly stressed, or want to feel and function 100 percent the next day.

A teenage patient I'll call Frances had frequent mood swings and emotional outbursts that caused problems with her family, school, and social life. Her symptoms were especially severe when she had too many sweets and didn't get enough sleep. Frances had been tentatively diagnosed with ADHD or manic depression and prescription medication was recommended.

Her mother brought her in for natural health care, hoping for a non-drug solution to her problems. Over time, Frances learned that she could turn her symptoms on and off by her lifestyle habits. A healthier diet, regular exercise, sufficient rest, and whole food supplementation helped transform her into a happy young lady who can deal with life's challenges without going ballistic.

Excessive amounts of sugar can have devastating physical and mental effects on certain people who, in turn, create a significant societal impact. Several mass murderers lived on pop and sugar laden junk foods. Too much sugar may have been the "last straw" in these and others who were already precariously imbalanced.

For all these reasons, eat white sugar products *sparingly* only if and when your body can handle the stress.

For more information about why you should avoid or minimize sugar, read: *Lick the Sugar Habit and Suicide* by Sugar by Nancy Appleton PhD.; *Sweet and Dangerous* by John Yudkin MD.; *Body, Mind, and Sugar* by E.M. Abrahamson MD; *Psychodietetics* by Cheraskin and Ringsdorf; *Sugar Blues* by William Dufty; *Low Blood Sugar and You and Psycho-Nutrition* by Carton Fredericks PhD; *Nutrition and Physical Degeneration* by Weston Price DDS; *Empty Harvest* by Bernard Jensen DC and Mark Anderson. Check the website at ***ppnf.org*** to learn more about pioneering work by Weston Price DDS and Francis Pottenger MD.

Whole Food Nutritional Supplements

Nutritional supplements are not a substitute for a healthy diet. However, *whole food supplements* are wise since nutrient values of foods have decreased due to topsoil deterioration; agribusiness use of pesticides, herbicides, and genetically modified seeds; pollution; and food processing, transport and storage practices. Many people also need additional nutrients due to deficiencies, prescription drug side effects, health problems, activity levels, and stress.

Because of these factors, even a healthy person with a consistently optimal diet needs good supplementation. Besides, how many people eat very well most of the time? For example, folic acid is most abundant in liver, kale, asparagus, beet greens, wheat bran, endive, spinach, and turnips. How often do you eat these foods? Getting optimal nutrition with the real food way of eating and *whole* food supplements makes sense.

Ensure that your nutritional supplements come from organically raised whole food sources. Whole food nutritional products are *highly bioavailable,* that is, easily used by the body. They also contain the *entire spectrum* of nutrients and cofactors as nature provided.

Why are these so important? As Royal Lee DDS, founder of the first whole food supplement company *Standard Process,* said: "The primary cause of disease isn't germs, genes, or toxins. It's malnutrition."

Here's one example: *real vitamin C* from food sources is a complex of several nutrients including ascorbic acid, organic copper, P factors, bioflavonoids, etc. Many cheap 'vitamin C' supplements are just synthetic ascorbic acid; other brands add a little rose hips thrown in so they can call it 'natural'.

Your body can function best when consuming the entire range of nutrients in the right amounts and forms that *occur naturally.*

Nutraceutical supplements – the kind that commercials advertise and most stores sell – contain high doses of synthetically derived nutrients. They are fractionated, that is, contain only a few nutrients versus hundreds found in whole foods. They also often contain *chemical coloring,* for example, yellow dye #2 or red dye #4. Who cares what color a supplement is? And who wants the added toxins?

Nutraceuticals are less expensive because they are synthesized in a laboratory from chemicals or unnatural sources like coal tar. Most of the ingredients in these commercial supplements come from pharmaceutical companies. They are not as dangerous as medical drugs, but high levels of synthetic vitamins are foreign to the body and potentially harmful.

Several university studies investigating the effects of isolated vitamins like A and E had to be halted because of increased morbidity (illness) and mortality (death) rates in the groups receiving treatment.

Taking commercial sources of supplements is also a waste of money because your body often *can't dissolve them.* Workers at water treatment plants and portable toilet businesses clean vast amounts of undissolved supplements from the filters. The brand names on these highly advertised but nutritionally bankrupt products are sometimes still legible.

Other products don't dissolve because they were never intended to be eaten. Calcium carbonate, for example, commonly comes from limestone or sea shells. There may be calcium in these supplements but can your body use it? In one study, only 5% of the calcium in popularly used products was actually absorbed.

To recap, most supplements sold in stores are:

- ***synthetic:*** *made from chemicals, not whole foods*
- ***fractionated:*** *contain just a few vitamins and minerals instead of the broad spectrum of hundreds of nutrients*
- ***high dose:*** *instead of lower doses in the right proportions as found in nature*
- ***poorly absorbed:*** *not usable or even recognizable by the body*

The *Standard Process* company has been the gold standard for whole food supplements since 1929. Their supplements are easily digested and used by the body. The plant sources are organically grown in rich topsoil, then concentrated via cold processing to maintain the vitality of enzymes and nutrients. The organ tissues that provide small amounts of essential nutrients come from animals raised and processed healthfully and humanely.

What Supplements Should You Take?

(**Note:** Moderate varieties the supplements mentioned are from *Standard Process* and can only be obtained from a licensed health care practitioner or via Patient Direct. Contact my office at *center@radiant101.com* if you do not have a local resource. At this time, whole food supplements can only be shipped to the U.S. fifty states and Puerto Rico because of import regulations. Visit *StandardProcess.com* to learn more about these products and evaluate ones from other companies.)

In the past, many health care practitioners used a one-size-fits-all approach to nutritional supplementation. More clinicians now recognize the importance of a *personalized or designed supplement regimen.* This objectively indicates the specific products a person needs and in what amounts. In the hands of a skilled evaluator, this is state-of-the-art nutritional testing and treatment.

To learn more, see the *Natural Health Care* section of this book. Many *people have healed themselves* of severe mental and physical ailments using these nutrition-based healing approaches.

Most patients initially need a *therapeutic regimen* of specific nutrients to counteract deficiencies of the entire body or certain organs. Once these deficiencies have been addressed, the body can often restore normal functioning. After that, a few *wellness supplements* cover many nutritional bases and help keep people well.

Wellness supplements include *Catalyn* (multivitamin and mineral), *Cod Liver Oil* or *Tuna Omega Oil* (essential fatty acids and vitamins

D and F), and *Trace Minerals B12.* Women, rapidly growing children, and men with muscle spasms often need *Calcium Lactate* and perhaps *Magnesium Lactate* and *Cataplex F.*

Three other common areas for supplement need are stomach acid, digestive enzymes, and intestinal flora.

Normal levels of *stomach acid* are needed for proper food and supplement breakdown and absorption. *Low levels* of gastric acid are common in people over age 40 and very common after age 60. Yes, contrary to what drug commercials may lead you to believe, most people have *too little acidity* in their gastric juices, not too much.

Causes of this condition called *hypochloridia* include: nutritional deficiencies, for example, of salt; poor function of key organs such as the stomach and pituitary gland; drinking too much fluid with meals; improper food combining; eating too much at once; poor diet with too much sugar and fat; and acid-blocking prescription drugs or antacids.

If you get indigestion after eating or taking whole food supplements, you may need additional stomach acidity from a product like *Zypan* that contains betaine hydrochloride.

Digestive enzymes are needed to break down food and assist optimal digestion. Enzymes are found in living foods, especially pineapple, papaya, raw organic honey, raw cow and goat milk products, raw fruits and vegetables, and certain herbs. Some people need a product like *Multizyme* to restore normal enzyme levels in the gastrointestinal or GI tract.

Probiotics provide normal flora for healthy digestive tract functioning. An imbalance between 'good' and 'bad' bacteria and yeast can occur due to poor nutrition, antibiotic use, and other factors. An overgrowth of bad flora and/or deficiency of good flora can cause many common physical and mental symptoms.

The GI tract produces as many neuropeptides—protein messengers that aid nervous system communication—as does the brain. That's why GI imbalances can cause mental symptoms such as depression, brain fog and anxiety as well as excess gas, diarrhea, and constipation.

People may need one or more normal flora products to restore balanced microorganism levels and wellness. *Prosynbiotic, Lactenz,* and *Lactic Acid Yeast* are three Standard Process products for this need.

This information may seem overwhelming initially, but it's not that complicated. Learning this information can be remarkably life-changing. Once you understood the principles involved, you can prevent and reverse many common symptoms that plague you and your loved ones.

For more information, read: *Why Your Doctor Offers Nutritional Supplements* by Stephanie Selene Anderson; *The Real Truth about Vitamins and AntiOxidants* by Judith DeCava MS, LNC; and resources from ***SeleneRiverPress.com*** and ***StandardProcess.com***.

Real Food Way of Eating: Healing Phase

This approach is needed as a person addresses significant health problems, overweight, and imbalances. Strictly follow these guidelines for **only 90 days**. Most people can then graduate to the *Wellness Phase* that involves eating healthfully 90 95% of the time. (That means you can occasionally eat small amounts of whatever you want.)

This phase is very low in sugar. Why? Excess sugar can cause overweight, inflammation, insulin resistance, metabolic syndrome, increased cholesterol and triglyceride levels, diabetes, and increased microorganism growth. Heavy metals and chemicals reside inside these microorganisms and are also stored in fat. Excess carbs – as you know – are converted to sugar that, in turn, may be stored as fat.

That's why I recommend green powders, protein powders, and protein bars from *Standard Process, Garden of Life,* or *Vibrant Living.* The whole food supplements listed are from *Standard Process* and

MediHerb. Visit websites of these companies to learn more about the content and quality of their products. That will allow you to evaluate brands that may be good but I just don't know about.

Guidelines:

- *Eat fresh and unprocessed foods that are chemical-free, nonGMO, and healthfully raised.*
- *Read labels and AVOID the following: sugar, wheat, soy, corn, hydrogenated oils, artificial sweeteners, and high fructose corn syrup. Also AVOID meat, eggs, or dairy from unhealthily raised sources*
- ***If it's not on the list below, don't eat it for 90 days.***

Protein: 2 servings per day

- *Meat: wild caught fish; pasture-raised chicken, turkey, beef, or buffalo; wild game. No cured meats. Serving size is the size and thickness of your palm.*
- *Eggs: 2-3 whole eggs plus 1-2 egg whites for more protein*
- *Dairy: from certified raw or organic, flash pasteurized pasture-raised sources*
- *Protein powder from plant or whey for smoothies*
- *Protein bars with plant or whey sourced protein and low carbs*
- *Vitality Drink (see below) for plant and seed sources of protein*
- *Grain and legume combination for complementary amino acids*

Note: Use rice, almond, or coconut milk but not soy

Vegetables: unlimited amounts allowed, but at least 4-6 servings per day

- *eat vegetables raw, juiced, steamed, lightly sautéed, or in soups*
- *avoid the starchy (high sugar) varieties: white potatoes, corn, yams, peas*
- *eat at least one raw vegetable salad per day*
- *green powder with a variety of grasses, vegetables, and sprouts*

For dressing: use cold pressed oil with apple cider vinegar or lemon juice; homemade with organic ingredients; or good brands such as Haines, Annie's, and Newman's

Raw Nuts & Seeds: 1 2 servings per day of RAW almonds, pecans, walnuts, or macadamia nuts; chia, hemp, pumpkin, sunflower, sesame, and flax seeds. These are best eaten after soaking for 20 minutes. Visit ***TheRawtarian.com*** for additional information about sprouting.

Healthy Fats: healthy fats and oils: pasture-raised butter, ghee, coconut butter, avocado, eggs; olive, grape seed, walnut, sesame, safflower, and coconut oils

Legumes: adzuki, pinto, black, garbanzo, fava, edamame, soy, red kidney, and lima beans; black eyed peas, lentils. Dried organic legumes soaked overnight before cooking are better than canned. Legumes are also great sprouted.

Grains: 0 1 serving of grains or legumes per day depending on your health status and weight loss goals. Organic sprouted grain bread and cereal. Wheat-free grains, crackers and pasta from brown rice, quinoa, amaranth, or millet.

Fruit: 1 serving per day of low glycemic varieties: raspberries, strawberries, blueberries, blackberries, and Granny Smith apples

Sweeteners: 0-1 serving per day of stevia, xylitol or agave; no artificial sweeteners

Condiments: natural herbs and spices; Borsari and Celtic Sea Salt; no or low sugar brands of mustard, catsup and meat sauces

Beverages: pure water with lemon and lime added if desired; herbal teas; 1-2 cups of organic coffee or tea per day

Health Drinks: two blended drinks that I highly recommend are described below. These require a *VitaMix* or similar high powered blender that pulverizes the foods into a drink. The recipes given are for me: a 185 pound active mesomorph who exercises six days a week. You may want to reduce or increase the quantities of each ingredient depending on your weight, body type, weight loss goals, and activity levels.

- ***Vitality Drink:*** *a nutrient-dense combination with extraordinary energy and satiety. Here's my current recipe: 42 ounces pure water, 1 scoop of raw green powder, ½ small lemon, 1 stalk celery, ½ TB pomegranate powder, 4 inch section cucumber, ½ tsp. Sea or Himalayan salt, 3 Hawaiian spirulina tablets, 5 chlorella tablets, handful of spinach leaves, 1 TB pumpkin seeds, 1 TB sunflower seeds, 1 TB hemp seeds, 1 TB chia seeds, 1 TB black sesame seeds, 1 large carrot, 1/4 medium beet, one small apple, few sprigs of parsley, 2 inch piece of turmeric and ginger, handful of sunflower or kale sprouts, dash or two of black pepper. Makes 64 ounces.*
- ***Protein Smoothie:*** *32 ounces of water, 6 8 ounces of berries (blue berries, black berries, strawberries, or raspberries), 40 grams of protein powder, 1 TB flax seeds, 1 TB Calcifood Powder, 1 tsp. Calcium Lactate powder, handful of raw nuts, and ice. Makes about 64 ounces.*

Other drinks: these are designed to help you lose weight, increase your energy and mental clarity, and heal your endocrine system:

1. ***Breakfast Butter Tea/Coffee:*** *16-ounces hot water, serving tea or coffee, ½ true TB pasture-raised butter, 1 TB MCT oil OR ½ true TB raw organic coconut butter. This helps your body burn fat as its primary fuel source instead of glucose. That, in turn, can help your pancreas and liver heal and stabilize blood sugar levels throughout the day.*

1. ***Bedtime Butter Tea:*** *If you crave sweets at bedtime or have insomnia due to hunger, sip before bedtime: 10 ounces pure water, relaxing herbal tea, cinnamon or other spice, ½ true tsp raw honey, and 1 true TB butter or coconut butter.*

2. ***Modified 24 hour Fast:*** *once per week, consume only pure water, green powder, and juiced vegetables for breakfast and lunch.*

Note: consult your integrative medicine doctor and natural health care practitioners before using #1-3 if there is any concern about your blood sugar or other health condition.

The real food way of eating is how humans have always eaten until food industries destroyed nutrients and brainwashed consumer choices via advertising.

You now have a choice to make. What is more important to you? Eating the way that is more convenient and temporarily stimulates your taste buds and brain that are addicted to sugar and chemicals? Or making some changes and feeling happy, healthy and energetic again?

Real Food Way of Eating: Wellness Phase

When you are healthy and have reached your desired weight, you are ready for the wellness phase. The keys? Eat the Healing Real Food Way of Eating 90-95% of the time.

This lifetime way of eating follows the 90-Day Healing approach 90-95% of the time and allows you to enjoy an occasional sweet or junk food. Your body will let you know if you are eating too much junk too often. Once you feel great and happy nearly all the time, you can use that yardstick to monitor whether you are sufficiently following dietary and other laws of health. If your health status and weight allow, you can now have:

- ***Occasional starchy carbs:*** *white potatoes, corn, yams, peas*
- ***Two servings of grains or legumes*** *per day*
- ***Two servings of fruit*** *per day, primarily low and moderate with occasional high glycemic varieties*
- ***Dairy products*** *if your weight and health status tolerate them*
- ***Healthier snacks*** *two or three times a week: fruit sweetened cookies; dark chocolate with 70 percent or higher cocoa content; popcorn; muffins or fruit cobbler made with gluten-free grains, nuts, fruit, and natural sweeteners; potato or sweet potato chips;*

cold processed whole food bars with about 18 grams of plant or whey protein and 5 net grams of carbs.

- ***Junk food rarely:*** *pizza, ice cream, decadent dessert, etc. You'll feel worse, gain weight, and go backwards in your wellbeing if you eat too much too often.*

Again, if this way of eating sounds boring, just consider what is more important: feeling, looking *and being* your very best or eating whatever you want and being like the average person?

Howie, a forty-year-old ex-college athlete, was 55 pounds overweight and suffered with—I'm not exaggerating—25 different symptoms. After using the real food way of eating and whole food supplements for six months, he lost all the extra weight and all of his symptoms.

After just four months of following this program, Jim, a sixty-five-year-old retired factory worker, lost 40 pounds and felt more energy than he had in 20 years. His blood pressure, blood sugar, and cholesterol levels all returned to normal. At his next office visit, his medical doctor thought he had the wrong chart because all of Jim's lab values were normal. This is how it can be and should be.

What Do I Eat?

I am often asked what I eat. At age 64, I feel happy, healthy, and energetic almost all the time. When I don't, I can usually evaluate the cause and correct it. I weigh only seven pounds more than when I graduated from high school. My nutritional program is an integral part of all that.

The way of eating I'll described may seem boring or difficult to you. I love great tasting foods, but many years of eating healthfully have altered my definition of *what tastes good.* Almonds taste sweet, fresh berries are heavenly, and I love my health drinks. Most importantly, feeling great all the time is much more important than eating unhealthy foods that are sweet, fatty, processed, and convenient.

Except for occasional small servings, I avoid wheat, soy, sugar, and dairy products since those cause a day or two of depression, fatigue, brain fog, sinus drainage, and intestinal upset. I also avoid foods that aren't organic since those are chemically laden with pesticides and herbicides.

For over forty years I've refined my way of eating and enjoyed daily prayer, yoga, meditation, and regular time in nature. I have eaten a nutrient-dense semi-vegetarian diet for most of that time. Every aspect of my life is working wonderfully: great health, loving relationships, prosperity, meaningful lifework, inner peace, happiness, and a deep knowing that I am a forever being. All of those factors increase, balance, and upgrade my energy. As a result, I don't need the quantity of heavy foods, especially animal products, that I once did.

My whole food maintenance supplements from *Standard Process* include *Catalyn, Trace Minerals B12,* and *Cod Liver Oil.* I take *CardioPlus* and *Cyruta Plus* for my cardiovascular system, *Symplex M* for endocrine support, and *Cataplex B* and *Cataplex B12* because of my ovo-vegetarian diet. I feel satiated after less food because my body isn't always hungry for something else and searching for key nutrients that can't be found in devitalized foods.

I don't recommend completely switching to my way of eating overnight since it is such a big change for most people. However, I strongly encourage doing so if you desire to lose a significant amount of weight, heal yourself of serious symptoms or a named disease, or enjoy more vibrant living. Otherwise, consider incrementally moving in this direction.

Needless to say, the foods are healthfully raised with sustainable agriculture methods whenever possible. The foods are organic or beyond organic, fresh, GMOfree, chemical-free, and mostly raw. The term 'raw' means that the foods were not exposed to temperatures over 115 degrees Fahrenheit so nutrients, enzymes, and cofactors aren't devitalized or destroyed.

If I don't feel like having the vitality and protein drinks on a certain day, I eat meals from the Light Evening Meal list, but that rarely happens. I usually travel with my VitaMix so I can enjoy the drinks even while away from home.

Note: See Real Food Way of Eating: Healing Phase for drink recipes

First, Breakfast Butter Tea. (Satisfies me for 3 hours afterwards)

Then Vitality Drink (I drink these over a 4 hour period)

Next, Protein Smoothies (I drink these over a 4 hour period)

Light Evening Meal

- *Egg omelet, deviled eggs, or quiche 2 3 times per week with 2 whole eggs and 2 egg whites and sautéed vegetables—onion, tomato, spinach—cooked in olive or grapeseed oil. I add sea salt and ½ avocado for additional good fats.*
- *Gluten-free Middle Eastern, Asian, Indian, or other ethnic foods*
- *Yogurt from almond or coconut milk with fresh berries and nuts*
- *Steamed/sautéed vegetables with brown rice/noodles, or quinoa*
- *Soup with vegetables, grains and/or legumes*
- *Large mixed vegetable salad with nuts and fresh fruit*
- *Hummus or guacamole with glutenfree crackers or chips and sliced vegetables*
- *Trail mix with raw nuts, seeds, and a little sugar-free dried fruit*
- *Healthy protein bar with a handful of raw nuts*
- *Rice cakes or toasted Ezekiel bread with raw almond butter*
- *Gluten-free cereal with chopped nuts, berries, and almond or coconut milk*

Snacks:

- *Two times per week: healthier snacks listed under the* ***Maintenance Way of Eating,*** *usually dark chocolate or popcorn with butter and brewer's yeast. The popcorn is part of my dinner after a small salad.*

- *Rarely, a decadent dessert. I thoroughly savor several bites and usually that is enough. Just being able to have it helps me to usually not want it.*

Bedtime: *if hungry or want something sweet, a cup of Bedtime Butter Tea*

Living Foods

Fresh and raw *living foods* are more nutritious and a must for those desiring radiant wellness. Make fresh and raw fruits and vegetables, sprouted grains, and raw nuts and seeds at least one third of your food intake each day. This requires more time than picking up convenience food from a drive-through, but the extra effort is well worth it now and in the future.

Eating living foods also prevents food cravings and overeating in an attempt to obtain essential nutrients. You know how pregnant women can develop strange food cravings? That is, in part, the result of trying to fulfill nutritional needs. Cows and horses are the same way. They will eat a wooden fence if they don't have a salt lick and sufficient minerals in their feed.

That's one reason why so many people are so overweight. The nutrients their bodies are craving *can't be found* in junk and processed foods. So they keep grazing and going through one snack after another. Patients using the healing and wellness real food ways of eating are amazed that *they don't feel hungry all the time anymore.* They have much more energy, enjoy the taste of real food, and lose a lot of weight.

I'm not advocating eating all raw and fresh food, but most people can benefit by greatly increasing their intake of living foods. Even orthodox dieticians have long counseled that the nutritive value of food decreases when cooked, frozen, processed, or stored: fresh is best, frozen next, and canned is the least nutritious choice.

A Paul Harvey radio commentary best explains what I mean by living foods. A sunken ship was found after several centuries; among the ballast were various plant seeds that actually sprouted and grew when given the right conditions of soil, water, and sunlight. After hundreds of years, those seeds *still contained life-giving properties* to grow healthy plants.

There is a spark of life and creative energy in all living things. This life force or vital energy has long been recognized by other cultures: the Chinese called it *chi,* the people of India *prana,* in Japan *ki.*

Eating lots of raw foods requires a healthy digestive tract. If you suffer with impaired digestion or diverticulitis, you may need to eat blended, steamed or juiced vegetables. Steaming improves the availability of the nutrients and reduces the potential of irritation from uncooked fiber. Add a little sea salt to the broth from the steamer and sip, or use in soups to recover nutrients lost during cooking.

Various healing regimens use fasting, raw foods, fresh juices, whole food supplements, and other approaches to *help the body heal itself* of supposedly incurable diseases. Resources include:

- **Recipes for Longer Life** *by Ann Wigmore ND, founder of the Hippocrates Institutes*
- **Dr. Jensen's Juicing Therapy** *by Bernard Jensen DC, PhD.*
- **A Cancer Therapy—Results of 50 Cases** *by Max Gerson, MD.*
- *Books by N.W. Walker DSc, John Christopher ND, MH, and Dr. Herbert M. Shelton*
- **Eat to Live** *by Joel Fuhrman MD.*
- **The Miracle of Fasting and The Bragg Healthy Lifestyle** *by Paul Bragg (who was Jack LaLanne's teacher)*
- **The Hallelujah Diet** *by Rev. George Malkmus*
- **Power Juices, Super Drinks** *and other books by Steve Meyerowitz*

Raw Nuts and Seeds

Raw nuts and seeds are a good secondary source of protein, fats, and carbohydrates. Walnuts, pecans, almonds, and macadamia nuts and their nut butters are recommended unless you have an allergy to tree nuts. Use cashews minimally because of the oxalate content. Keep them refrigerated to keep them fresh.

Peanuts are actually legumes that grow underground. As such, they are susceptible to mold and fungal growth. Peanuts are much more likely to cause allergic reactions than tree nuts. Peanuts do have nutritional benefit, however. If you eat peanut butter, make sure it's unprocessed and without sugar.

Raw chia, flax, sesame, hemp, sunflower and *pumpkin seeds* provide lots of nutrients, taste and health benefits. Raw seeds can be eaten alone or sprinkled on salads, soups, pasta and rice dishes. They can be added to muffins, warm or cold cereal, and yogurt. Seeds can be ground up in raw bars, smoothies, and veggie burgers.

Juicing and Sprouting

Juicing and sprouting are simple ways to enjoy lots of living foods. Machines made by *Champion* and Jack LaLanne's *Power Juicer* separate the juice from the pulp. Others, such as the *VitaMix,* grind up the entire fruit or vegetable and provide even more nutrients. Juices purchased in stores are often made from concentrate, are acidic, and have gone through processing that kills nutrients.

Juicing does take some time so you could juice enough for a week, then quickly freeze 16-ounce portions in plastic cups with sealed lids. This isn't as good as totally fresh, though, so juice daily if your schedule allows or your health needs require it.

Sprouting is another excellent way to obtain living foods. Only a wide-mouth jar, nylon net or cheesecloth, and a rubber band are needed. If nuts, seeds and grains have been cooked, roasted, or otherwise exposed to high temperatures, they will not sprout. This is the acid test of whether a food is living or dead. Sprouts are an excellent source of vitamins, minerals, enzymes, and chlorophyll.

Put three tablespoons of nuts, seeds or grains in a jar and wash them well with water. Drain and thoroughly shake out the water through the screen over the jar's opening. Put the jar on its side after shaking the seeds around so they are distributed on the lower side. Cover the jar with a hand towel to speed sprout growth. Rinse and drain the seeds twice each day. Drain off all the water, but don't let them dry out.

When the sprouts reach the size you like best, put them in full sunlight until tiny green leaves appear. Tightly cover, store in the refrigerator and *eat within three to four days.* Use these tasty sprouts in your salads, stir fry vegetables, Mexican, Asian, and other dishes. Alfalfa, sunflower, mung bean, lentil, and wheat berries are most commonly used, but you can sprout any raw nut, seed, or grain.

Juicing and sprouting will become common practices as more people realize the importance of raw, fresh living foods. You can't vibrantly support a living system on dead and devitalized foods. For additional information about sprouting and juicing, read books by authors cited in the *Living Foods* section above.

Food Combining Principles

Proper food combining principles have long been endorsed by many natural health experts. Try it for just 60 days and see if you feel and function better. Improper food combining can contribute to fatigue, gas, constipation, diarrhea, rectal itching, indigestion, and other symptoms. Try remembering who you are and why you're here when you're bombarded with those lovely symptoms. Proper food combining is especially important for those with sensitive or stressed digestive systems, or existing illnesses.

In short, this approach claims that *heavy proteins and starches don't digest well together.* Heavy proteins include any meat, but also eggs and dairy products to a lesser degree. Starches include baked goods, grains, potatoes, beans, legumes, pasta, and pastries. Non-starchy vegetables can digest equally well with either protein or starches.

Eating heavy proteins and starches, such as meat and potatoes or bread, together makes efficient digestion difficult. The result can be incomplete digestion with partial putrefaction of proteins and fermentation of starches.

Some recommend the 80/20 rule of food combining *if you are healthy.* That is, you can combine a small amount of carbohydrates (20 percent) with a meal that is 80 percent protein or vice-versa. Examples are Ezekiel bread (carbs) with eggs (protein), or corn chips (carbs) with cheese and beans (contain carbs and protein.)

A properly combined meal can leave the stomach in about three hours whereas an improperly combined one may take six or more hours. Trying to digest and dispose of an improperly combined meal requires extra energy output by the body. That's one reason why the average person experiences after meal fatigue, low energy levels in general, and a host of gastrointestinal symptoms.

My personal experience convinces me that proper food combining principles are wise. After an improperly combined meal, I can tell by the feeling of fullness and belching that my stomach is still digesting five to six or more hours. I'll spare you the details of what happens twenty-four hours later as an improperly combined meal is eliminated. These symptoms never happen after a properly combined meal.

Eating fruit properly is another principle in food combining. Simply put, it's best to eat fruit alone or leave it alone. (Blending fruit with protein powders in smoothies is usually OK since the liquid moves quickly out of the stomach.) Fruit is easily digested and, when eaten alone, exits from the stomach into the small intestine in about 20 minutes.

If fruit is eaten with or immediately after other foods, however, it is blocked from its normal and rapid course of digestion. Fruit sugars then ferment and increase bacterial growth, gas production, and other undesirable symptoms.

This explains why some people think they can't tolerate eating fruit. Indigestion after improper food combining is nature's way of complaining. Fruit is a perfect food when eaten alone or 20 minutes before other food. Since properly combined meals take 3 to 4 hours to leave the stomach, wait that long after a meal before eating fruit again.

You don't have to get too obsessive about this. A small amount of fruit won't cause much trouble with most foods. Consider, though, how fruit sugars would get blocked when eaten after a heavy meal of salad, steak, baked potato, and roll.

The next proper food combining recommendation is to *avoid drinking excess fluid with your meal.* Gastric juices of a specific strength aid optimal digestive efficiency. If you drink too much fluid during your meal, your digestive juices are diluted and weakened. Drink some water 15 minutes before a meal, then wait an hour or more after a meal before drinking much fluid. You can, of course, have a few sips of water during and after the meal if needed.

Finally, *eat a lighter dinner earlier in the evening.* You'll likely experience nighttime indigestion, especially if you are middle-aged or older, after eating a large dinner late in the evening. A large dinner is also more likely to be converted to fat since you are less active afterwards. If your health and body weight are good, you can enjoy two evening snacks per week as a special treat.

For more information about food combining, read *Gut Solutions* by Brenda Watson, ND and Leonard Smith MD; *Food Combining and Digestion* by Steve Meyerowitz; and *Food Combining Made Easy* by Herbert M. Shelton.

Breastfeeding

Breastfeeding is the vastly superior approach for both nutritionally and emotionally raising babies. Mother's breast milk—not cow or soy milk or technologically concocted formula—is nature's perfect food for human babies. Newborns should be breastfed exclusively for at least six months before adding *healthy* solid foods and nursed until the baby naturally weans.

One huge reason to do this is to prevent food allergies. In *Hidden Food Allergies,* Braly and Holford state that food allergies often occur when infants are fed anything other than breast milk. Their digestive systems are designed to process only one food—mother's breast milk.

Anything else—cow's milk, soy milk, or other formulas—may be mistaken as foreign invaders and rejected by the body's defense systems. This allergic reaction can generalize toward other foods and body cells, thus the increase in autoimmune diseases.

Breastfeeding gives babies the perfect start with optimal nutrients, natural antibodies, maternal bonding, emotional security, cranial bone alignment, and facial muscle development. For more information, contact your local Le Leche League and read *The Womanly Art of Breastfeeding.*

Nutrition for Youngsters

When your infant is ready for solid food, use a food strainer to produce healthy baby food. Lightly steam fresh vegetables, run through a strainer, and watch your baby enjoy broccoli, carrots, cauliflower and potatoes. Feed your little one *gluten-free whole grains* such as mashed brown rice, quinoa, amaranth or millet.

When they are ready for more protein, feed mashed or ground up *pasture-raised* eggs, chicken and turkey. As a healthy treat, use different fruits such as bananas, apples, kiwi, pears and melon. You can be assured this food is fresh, nonGMO, and unadulterated by pesticides, herbicides, and other chemicals.

Healthy and organic brands of commercially produced baby foods will do in a pinch, but there is no substitute for fresh whole foods. Vitamins, enzymes, and other micronutrients necessary for vital health are sensitive to temperature, light, and storage times.

High temperature cooking, freezing, packaging and storage cause fresh food to lose nutrients. That's why a healthy way of eating for children contains mashed, lightly steamed, and freshly juiced vegetables and pureed raw fruits.

As children grow older, their diets are more difficult to control. Ellyn Satter RD, ACSW, author of *Child of Mine: Feeding with Love and Good Sense,* counsels parents to avoid forcing children to eat healthy foods. Instead, she says, teach them by example and offer healthy alternatives. Keep only healthy food and nutritious snacks in the house so family members aren't tempted by unhealthy junk foods.

In time, children will learn to enjoy the taste of nutritious foods.

Remember that their stomachs are small and their metabolisms high. That's why children function better with more frequent but smaller meals and healthy snacks throughout the day.

Control your child's exposure to TV programs that advertise unhealthy junk foods. By age 18, the average child has watched 15,000 hours of TV versus spending 13,000 hours in school. Those TV hours include 350,000 commercials, many of which advertise heavily sugared and junk food products.

Send a nutritious home-packed lunch with your child to school most of the time. Years ago, I joined my daughters for lunch at school and was appalled at the menu: salami and baloney on white bread, a pickle, potato chips, apple sauce, milk, and a cookie. Any living or fresh foods in that meal?

This is the typical SAD (Standard American) meal with too much fat, sugar, salt, and processed foods with no fresh fruits or vegetables. Parents, work with the PTA and food service manager to ensure healthier lunches.

Children are born with a potential for optimal physical growth, mental development, immunity to disease, and longevity. The quality of a child's diet—especially during the prenatal and early childhood period—influences whether or not that potential will be expressed.

Recently, a mother brought in her fourteen-year-old daughter who was suffering with a long list of symptoms: depression, alternating constipation and diarrhea, sinus problems, nervousness, insomnia and more. They had been to a medical doctor who couldn't find anything wrong.

My evaluation showed that her immune system was imbalanced and she had an overgrowth of yeast and bacteria in her GI tract. I recommended the real food way of eating and whole food supplements to help her body heal itself.

When I presented the report of findings, the mother turned to her daughter and asked, "Is this something you want to do?" The daughter didn't, in part, because would have to eat less junk food. So they didn't start treatment.

Parents, don't try to be cool or a best friend. Be a good parent. Who else is going to fill that role for your child? That fourteen-year-old didn't know what was best for her and will likely suffer even more in the future because of her mother's failure to look out for her.

I know that busy parental schedules make it difficult to attend to nutritional details, but – in both the short and long term – the extra effort is well worth your children being healthier, happier, and better behaved. They grow up so quickly. Please provide them with the best nutritional start so they can fulfill their amazing potentials.

Nutritional Needs for Mothers

Karla, a thirty-eight-year-old mother who had recently given birth to her second child, came into my office. She had been a chiropractic patient for many years so I could tell something wasn't right with her. When I inquired, she broke down crying and admitted that she had been extremely depressed, nervous and exhausted. She couldn't focus mentally, didn't sleep well and was planning to kill herself. Her medical doctor recommended antidepressants, but those only made her feel worse due to several side effects.

I explained to Karla that *postpartum symptoms* were common, especially for mothers after two or more pregnancies whether those went full term or not. The developing and nursing baby pulls many nutrients from the mother's body. If these are not replaced correctly, and they seldom are, the mother's physical and mental health goes downhill from there.

After working with many thousands of patients in hospitals, mental health centers and private practice, I've taken histories on many women who reported that their health spiraled steadily downward after one or more pregnancies. "Ever since my second baby," they say, "I've never been the same."

After childbirth, women may be advised to continue taking a prenatal vitamin, but—as you now know—those are *synthetic* (made from chemicals, not whole foods), *fractionated* (contain just a few vitamins and minerals instead of the broad spectrum of nutrients found in nature), *high dose* (instead of lower doses as found in nature) and poorly absorbed (not usable or even recognizable by the body.) Most supplements bought in stores or pharmacies are like this.

Fortunately, we caught Karla's problem before she made a poor decision from her imbalanced state of mind. Her brain and adrenal or stress glands needed assistance. Within a few weeks of taking a personalized program of whole food supplements, she was back to her normal self. She now enjoys her family, her job, and life in general – just like she used to.

Please share this information with mothers of all ages. Some women are physical and emotional wrecks due to decades of nutritional deficiencies. The more pregnancies a woman has, the more likely she is to suffer with nutritional deficiencies. These symptoms may occur soon after the pregnancy ends or may take years to show up.

Doctors who don't understand the impact of nutritional imbalances may think these women are hysterical psychiatric cases. The ensuing downhill slide affects everyone: mother, children, and significant others. Fortunately, this problem is easily prevented and treated.

Children of nutritionally deficient women also often suffer from nutritional deficiencies. Think about it. If a mother is already low in key nutrients after previous pregnancies, the developing fetus doesn't have the usual stockpile to access. There's not much extra food in the pantry, so to speak. In my experience, children or teenagers with a lot of symptoms are often not firstborn.

Offending Foods

As I know very well from personal experience, offending foods can cause many serious physical and mental symptoms. I was nearly fifty years old before figuring out that my body does not tolerate wheat, dairy, corn, soy and sugar. Do you know how many processed foods those five are in?

I suffered with many symptoms that really were clues from my body that it didn't like those foods. Those symptoms hurt the quality of my life as a person, family member, friend, doctor, and teacher. I was often *good to great,* but not always *outstanding* as is possible.

Now I enjoy the real food way of eating 95 percent of the time and can occasionally tolerate eating a little bit of those foods. Avoiding offending foods is one reason I feel happy, healthy and energetic almost all of the time.

That's why I'm so passionate about getting this basic wellness information out to as many people as possible. Children shouldn't have to suffer so much nor should adults have to search high and low for solutions to their health problems.

In this brief overview, I will use the terms 'food allergies' and 'offending foods' synonymously. Both describe the body's way of telling you that it doesn't like a particular food. There are numerous factors involved: type of food, quality of food, general health of the person, elimination habits, genetic predisposition, and more.

For example, were the tomatoes you ate chemical-free or not? Was the beef pasture raised with grass as its primary feed or corn fed? Was the milk processed and from pen raised cows that received hormones and antibiotics? People may be allergic to eggs from commercially raised hens, but not to those from pasture raised birds.

People with wheat allergies may not be affected by products from Europe that have not been subjected to herbicides, pesticides, and genetic modification. Read books and articles by Michael Pollan to learn more about this topic that is so important for the health of you and your family.

The *health status* of a person also affects what foods he or she is offended by or allergic to. For example, foods containing yeast (wine, beer, aged cheeses, bread, pretzels, cider) may be especially problematic for those with an overgrowth of yeast in their body. If a person's filtration organs (colon, liver, kidneys, spleen) are working poorly or are overwhelmed, a person may be sensitive to more foods than if those systems were functioning normally.

Offending foods can cause many serious physical and mental symptoms. Certain foods can trigger abnormal function, inflammatory changes, and autoimmune reactions that especially contribute to symptoms of the following systems:

- *gastrointestinal (diarrhea, constipation, bloating, excess gas)*
- *musculoskeletal (joint and muscle pain, stiffness, or cramping)*
- *brain and nerves (depression, brain fog, anxiety, panic, fatigue)*

Marshall Mandell MD – author of *Allergy, the Unrecognized Cause of Physical, Mental, and Psychosomatic Illness* – says that *processed foods* containing sugar and white flour are common triggers of food allergies. Canned foods offend more often than fresh sources.

The most common allergy producing foods are dairy products, wheat, yeast, eggs, sugar, corn and soy. Nonfat and low-fat varieties of cow's milk are especially troublesome because there's less fat to buffer casein, the allergy producing protein in milk. Allergies to *gluten*—found in wheat, rye, barley, oats, kamut, spelt and triticale—are also very common.

Nutritional experts are also increasingly questioning the benefits of soy because it's a very common allergy-provoking food, is difficult to digest, and often comes from chemically sprayed and genetically modified sources. In moderation, *fermented, organic, nonGMO soy products* – miso, natto, tempeh and tofu – are better tolerated than non-fermented soy products. Serving sizes are an issue as well. Asian cultures tend to use small amounts while those in Western cultures overdo it.

People are most familiar with *IgE allergies* that cause *immediate onset reactions* such as those experienced with allergies to peanuts. The symptoms are obvious and directly follow eating an offending food. As such, they are relatively easy to identify and avoid.

Much more common, however, are *IgG or delayed onset allergies.* Symptoms from this type of food allergy typically take about 48 hours to show up and may not always trigger a reaction. Thus, it's difficult to determine what foods caused what symptoms. Paradoxically, people are sometimes most offended by foods that they like and eat the most.

As discussed in *Hidden Food Allergies* by James Braly MD and Patrick Holford, identifying IgG food allergies is easier with current testing methods. They recommend a quantitative IgG ELISA food allergy test.

Other methods of identifying problematic foods are food rotation and elimination techniques as described in *How to Control Your Allergies* by Robert Forman PhD; *The McDougall Plan* by John McDougall MD; or *Is This Your Child?* by Doris Rapp MD.

After 30 days of eliminating a food, reintroduce it and see if there are immediate inflammatory responses such as rash, itching, burning eyes or sinus drainage. Next, wait two days to see if any bowel, mental or musculoskeletal symptoms arrive. If that food seems OK, add it to your diet but no more than three times per week. Then test another food until you've gone through the list of suspected food allergies.

A *nutrition based healthcare program* is a great way to evaluate and handle offending foods. (see *Natural Care* chapter)

These nutrition-based healing methods use muscle testing to detect stressors such as food allergies. Treatment includes avoiding offending foods for 90 days and perhaps taking digestive enzymes and/or betaine hydrochloride to facilitate elimination of food residues in the body.

By the way, environmental allergies (pet hair, dust, mold, pollen, grass and other unavoidable particles) are sometimes secondary allergies due to *primary food allergies.* Many clinicians have found that environmental allergies decrease or disappear when food allergies are addressed.

Healthy Sun Exposure

Among its other benefits, sunlight promotes production of vitamin D so I'm including this topic in the Diet section.

Current warnings against *excessive* sun exposure are based on justifiable concerns about skin cancer. Certainly you should avoid tanning booths, sunburns, and too much sun exposure—especially during midday hours.

However, cautions can be taken too far. *Adequate sun exposure* is necessary for optimal vitamin D production, energy, mood, immunity and healthy sleep patterns. There are probably other benefits that are not yet fully understood.

However, a growing number of doctors are calling for *prudent sun exposure.* University researchers have found that a moderate amount of time in the sun *without sunscreen* may help prevent diabetes, multiple sclerosis, rheumatoid arthritis, osteoporosis, heart disease, and even some cancers. The reason? A vitamin D deficiency can contribute to each of these conditions.

Recommended exposure times are about 30 minutes three times per week for fair skinned people and more for those with dark skin who don't produce vitamin D as efficiently. Sunscreen decreases the absorption of sun rays that produce vitamin D and should not be worn during these limited sunbathing times. In addition, many sunscreens contain unhealthy chemicals with harmful effects.

A Stanford University team of immunologists recently studied the question of healthy sun exposure. They found that melanoma patients with appropriate levels of daily sun exposure actually had *better survival rates* than patients who spent little or no time in the sun. Increased vitamin D levels apparently contributed to a stronger immune system that can protect patients from skin cancer. Doctors commenting on the research suggested 30 to 60 minutes of sun exposure per day.

In *The Protein Power Life Plan,* Michael Eades MD and Mary Eades MD discuss this topic in a chapter called *Sunshine Superman.* They agree that sensible sunshine exposure is vital and provide guidelines for length of exposure based on where you live and the time of day and year.

Other esteemed medical doctors such as Julian Whitaker, Mark Hyman, and Andrew Weil agree. A growing number of scientific studies support the practice of healthy sun exposure. Dr. Whitaker says that lower levels of sunlight in northern hemispheres during winter months are primarily responsible for the higher incidence of flu and colds. He recommends limited sun exposure and at least 4000 IU of vitamin D per day, *not flu shots,* to combat this.

Scientific evidence aside, think about it for a moment. Humans have historically lived outdoors and naturally were exposed to sunlight. They probably didn't lie out in the midday sun for hours, but some sun exposure was part of their lifestyle.

Obtaining adequate sun exposure isn't always possible in winter months. Insufficient sunlight can contribute to depression known as seasonal affective disorder (SAD), sleep disorders, and other circadian rhythm disorders. *Light therapy,* especially blue light technology, provides light absorbed by the eyes and skin to combat these conditions. These devices have been researched at universities and are especially useful for people who work night shift and suffer with depression.

General Information

How you eat is also very important. Eat slowly and in pleasant surroundings. Avoid eating when you're emotionally upset. Most importantly, *chew food thoroughly and don't overeat.* Incomplete digestion can result in foreign-appearing substances in the bloodstream. The body may then treat certain foods as recurring foreign invaders and develop allergic responses to them.

Digestion is like buttoning a long coat: if the first button is not aligned correctly, none of the other buttons will line up. Chewing your food completely is the first step required in a series of digestive processes. Without proper chewing, the other steps don't work correctly. The result? Low energy, indigestion, excess gas, constipation, diarrhea, and general poor health!

Eat a variety of foods instead of a limited number of foods over and over. This requires some creativity with recipes, but provides a much broader range of nutrients. Also refrain from using aluminum cookware and a microwave to cook or warm food.

Implement dietary modifications gradually. Change eating habits at your own pace so positive changes become permanent, not an overnight fad. *Be patient* as your body starts changing within. You may experience a cleansing crisis like a cold or flu as your body cleans itself internally. You may temporarily need more rest as your body uses the extra energy to heal and balance.

Giving Thanks

Blessing food before eating is an age old and transcultural custom.

Healthy foods are endowed with a spark of life. Prayer honors the food's life force that, in turn, allows you to live. When you understand what a miracle this process is, you appreciate this sacred process of alchemy.

In repeated studies, sensitive measurements have indicated that plants, eggs, and animal cells have *an awareness* of events happening around them. When they are killed or hurt, their electrical emanations are the human equivalent of a scream.

However, *when food is prayed over* before it is cooked or eaten, it shows a calm pattern instead of frenetic graph activity. One possible interpretation of this data is that *all life has consciousness.* Food may recognize its role in supporting life forms that are respectful and appreciative.

Teddy, in J.D. Salinger's *Nine Stories,* saw his sister drinking milk and realized it was "like pouring God into God." The animal or plant that you consume gave its energy for your sustenance. That life force becomes incorporated into your very being and thus lives on. Give thanks for the food that allows you to be your very best.

Eat Healthfully?

Anyone who regularly eats healthfully can attest to the many wonderful benefits that occur. It is one of the most important keys to radiant wellness.

Remember Ed, the fourteen-year-old boy that I mentioned in the introduction of this chapter? You'll recall that he had been diagnosed with Crohn's disease at age eight and suffered with bloody diarrhea ten to twelve times per day. He received orthodox medical treatment of drugs, including powerful steroids. With no improvement, his doctors were considering removing his colon and installing a permanent colostomy bag.

For a fourteen-year-old boy!

His medical doctors never recommended any dietary changes or other natural approaches to assist digestion and calm inflammation. Just drugs, then surgery.

Fortunately, someone told his family about holistic health care and they decided to try it. His history revealed that he ate lots of foods that commonly cause allergies: wheat, dairy products, corn, sugar, and pork.

He agreed to change his way of eating to remove these potentially offending foods.

I also started him on nutritional supplements to provide key nutrients, assist digestion, and decrease inflammation: a multivitamin mineral, probiotics, digestive enzymes, fish oil, and a formula for promoting intestinal health.

A spinal exam, x-rays, and video-fluoroscopic imaging revealed significant vertebral misalignment in the upper neck where the spinal cord exits the brain. Additional spinal malposition was seen in the lower back where nerves supply the intestines. I adjusted these vertebrae to ensure optimal nerve supply from the brain to gastrointestinal system.

Within a week, Ed was having only five to six episodes of diarrhea a day and no bleeding. In two weeks, his bowel movements were decreased to three a day and becoming more solid. Within three weeks, he was having two normal bowel movements a day.

At that point, he decided to celebrate with a meal containing wheat, dairy and sugar. The next day, he had bloody diarrhea. Ed and his family were then convinced about the relationship between nutrition and disease.

Three years after beginning treatment, he has two normal stools a day with no bleeding, cramping or pain. He doesn't take any medication. Ed sleeps throughout the night and can enjoy school without having to worry about running out of the classroom with severe diarrhea. No longer swollen from steroids, he has a newfound confidence and zest for life. His body can now handle an *occasional treat* or offending food without flairups.

Now you understand why optimal nutrition is so important. Like Ed, many people are suffering needlessly and living suboptimal lives when it can be so much better. Maybe they don't have a serious disease yet, but the quality of their lives still suffers.

Over the last forty years, I have worked with many dying and very ill patients. If they could do it over again, they always say, they would take better care of themselves. Please don't wait until you're in a crisis or it's too late. Take the time to educate yourself, improve your lifestyle habits, and enjoy the life you deserve.

Healthy nutrition can help you feel great every day, wake up excited about life and have exuberant energy. As an old Japanese saying counsels: "The best time to plant a tree is twenty years ago. The second best time is today." *Start today* with nutritional improvements to transform yourself into the vital, healthy, and energetic person you can be.

Watch the videos *Food, Inc., Knives Over Forks, Fast Food Nation,* and *Fat, Sick and Nearly Dead* to learn about problems created by poor nutrition and good solutions. I also recommend articles and videos by: Mark R. Anderson at ***SeleneRiverPress.com***; Weston Price DDS and Francis Pottenger MD at ***ppnf.org***; Royal Lee, DDS at ***DrRoyalLee.com***; and ***StandardProcess.com***.

Recommended books for healthy eating include: *Eating on the Wild Side* by Jo Robinson; *The Longevity Kitchen* by Rebecca Katz; *Real Food* by Nina Planck; *Good Calories, Bad Calories* by Gary Taubes; *The Protein Power Life Plan* by Michael Eades MD and Mary Eades MD; *The Schwarzbein Principle* by Diane Schwarzbein MD; *Good Foods/ Bad Foods* by Judith DeCava; *The Zone* by Barry Sears PhD; *In Fitness and in Health* by Philip Maffetone DC; and *The Blue Zones* books by Dan Buettner.

Suggested cookbooks include: *The Schwarzbein Principle Cookbook* and *The Schwarzbein Principle Vegetarian Cookbook* by Diana Schwarzbein MD; *Nourishing Traditions* by Sally Fallon and Mary Enig PhD; *The Healthy Kitchen* by Andrew Weil MD; *Vegetarian Times Complete Cookbook* by Vegetarian Times magazine; *The Real Food Cookbook* and *The Farmer's Market Cookbook* by Nina Planck.

Note: This information is not designed to diagnose or treat any disease or replace medical care. It is based on Dr. Pitstick's many years of professional training and experience in addition to views of other naturally-oriented physicians. His recommendations are not supported by large medical studies, especially those funded by the disease care and pharmaceutical industries.

———◆———

The Bottom Line

The most important points in the Diet chapter include:

1. *Follow the real food way of eating with pure water, fresh organic vegetables, fruits, raw nuts and seeds, legumes, eggs, and lean meat.*
2. *Eat in such a way that you feel energetic and light afterwards.*
3. *Avoid trans fats, white flour, and white sugar; minimize caffeine.*
4. *Eat sufficient healthy fats and protein, but moderate carbs.*
5. *Breastfeed babies until they wean naturally and feed children healthfully.*
6. *Use only excellent sources of whole food supplements.*
7. *Follow food combining and other natural hygiene principles.*
8. *Consider a nutrition-based or other food allergy testing method if unexplainable physical and mental symptoms persist.*
9. *Get healthy sun exposure, but not too much.*
10. *Give thanks for life-giving nutrition that helps you live fully.*

Action Steps for Optimal Nutrition

List two action steps you commit to starting within 30 days:

1. ______________________________
2. ______________________________

List two action steps you commit to starting within 60 days:

1. ______________________________
2. ______________________________

List two action steps you commit to starting within 90 days:

1. ______________________________
2. ______________________________

RADIANT

Inner Cleanse

Key #4
Inner Cleanse

Doris had only one bowel movement *per week,* drank very little water, and didn't exercise—and her body showed it. Only thirty seven years old, she experienced many health problems including heavy menstrual flows, chronic sinus, bloating, and fatigue. Despite regular hygiene, she also had blemishes, body odor, and bad breath.

Not very radiant.

After starting the real food way of eating, more water, light exercise, and chiropractic adjustments, her body began catching up with the waste removal load. At first, she developed diarrhea for a few days—a good thing considering her inner toxicity. Her various symptoms were gone within two months. She now has daily bowel movements, her sinuses are clear, and her periods are symptom free. She looks, acts, feels, and smells better!

Detoxification is necessary in the 21st century because of the abundance of excess chemicals, heavy metals, microorganisms, and other impurities in food, air, water, medicines, body care products, home and laundry cleaning products, building materials, etc. You can't totally escape that toxic load but can minimize it with inner cleanse practices.

These toxins especially impact the brain and are – in my opinion and that of many other holistic physicians – one reason for the increase in neuromuscular disorders, memory loss, and mental symptoms such as depression, ADD, and others.

Normally, waste products are routinely removed in five ways. These *primary eliminative routes* and their associated organs are:

1. *Bowel movements (intestines)*
2. *Urination (kidneys)*
3. *Sweating (sweat glands and skin)*
4. *Deep breathing (lungs)*
5. *Blood filtration (liver, spleen and kidneys)*

Some people might consider these topics gross, but internal cleansing mechanisms are nothing to be embarrassed about. Those who are uptight about these habits are more likely to 'hold it in' and become toxic. The long-term consequences of improper elimination are really gross so let's discuss each route in more detail.

Bowel Movements

Orthodox medical advice says it's OK to have only a few bowel movements per week, but natural health experts consider that to be wrong. *There's a big difference between what is common and what is healthy.* Many people suffer with constipation, but that doesn't mean it's normal.

Your bowels should move easily at least twice a day. The 'poop' should be large in size and medium brown in color. Although it shouldn't smell like fresh flowers, your bowel movement should not have an awful odor. Straining out hard, dark, and horrible smelling rabbit pellets a few times per week isn't healthy.

Let's talk about intestinal gas for a moment. Everyone has some because it's a by-product of digestion. However, excess and overly foul gas and uncomfortable abdominal bloating are not normal. Something is imbalanced in your digestive system if you have frequent gas in large amounts and it causes people to run away in horror.

Regular bowel habits are assisted by exercise, healthy diet, adequate water intake, and a proper nerve supply. Following the urge to eliminate as soon as possible is another key. Your bowel movement rhythm can be thrown off if you hold it in.

If necessary, other approaches that can improve bowel movements include: (more details about #1 – 6 discussed in *Diet* section)

1. ***Healthy bacteria and yeast****—normal flora—to colonize the intestinal tract and aid optimal digestion*
2. ***Digestive enzymes*** *to assist breakdown of all food groups*
3. ***Hydrochloric acid*** *to improve digestion in the stomach*
4. ***Fish or flax oil*** *to lubricate the inner intestinal walls and assist optimal gut function*
5. ***Purification/detox programs,*** *for example, from Standard Process*
6. ***Nutrition-based evaluation*** *since anything can cause anything. For example, thyroid imbalance can negatively affect the kidneys and that, in turn, can cause colon dysfunction.*
7. ***Fiber supplements*** *in capsules, powders, or bars*
8. ***Colonics*** *by a certified colon hydrotherapist*
9. ***Bellows breathing assists*** *the movement of wastes through the intestinal tract. While seated, breathe deeply and with moderate forcefulness for a few minutes. Breathe fairly quickly but not so much that you get light-headed. Let your abdomen relax and bulge outward* ***while inhaling.*** *Pull your abdominal muscles in and up* ***while exhaling.***

Urination

If you drink sufficient water, you should urinate periodically throughout the day and once during the night. As mentioned, one guideline for water intake in ounces per day is your body weight in pounds divided by two or three.

Your urine should be a pale straw color and should not have a disagreeable odor. As with bowel movements, listen to your body's signals and urinate as soon as possible when the urge hits.

The kidneys produce urine by filtering the blood. Good kidney function is assisted by optimal water intake, nutrition, nerve supply, yoga postures that tone and massage internal organs, and proper hygiene to avoid urinary tract infections.

Sweating

Sweating eliminates wastes through pores and is an essential part of inner cleanliness. Our ancestors sweated by working hard and being in temperature extremes. Various cultures, Native American sweat lodges and Scandinavian saunas, for example, have long recognized the benefits of sweating.

You can sweat regularly by using the following methods:

- ***Exercise***
- ***Saunas:*** *infrared sauna is the most effective and requires lower temperatures than other types*
- ***Hot baths:*** *either in your bathtub or a hot tub. Soak for 30 minutes or more at a sufficient temperature to cause sweating. Salt water spas are best; avoid chlorinated products. Use a whole house filter to minimize chlorine in your bathtub.*
- ***Steam baths:*** *also very effective in producing a cleansing sweat*
- ***Sunbathing*** *in moderation, as discussed*

Since your skin is the eliminative organ involved in sweating, here are some recommendations for healthy skin:

1. ***Use healthy soaps, oils and lotions*** *from natural products. These should not include chemicals, dyes, and artificial fragrances.*
2. ***Skin brush,*** *using a dry brush or loofa, to remove dead cells and waste products that emanate from the pores*

3. ***Use whole food or herbal cleanses*** *that help detox and cleanse skin, pores, and associated glands*

4. ***Use natural deodorants*** *that don't expose your body to chemicals and heavy metals. The armpits have a rich supply of sweat glands, blood vessels, and lymphatic tissue that can absorb toxins. Especially avoid antiperspirant deodorants that contain aluminum, dyes, and harmful chemicals.*

5. ***Don't wear any deodorant*** *when it doesn't matter if you have a little body odor. Avoid deodorant when you exercise so your sweat glands and pores can eliminate wastes.*

Our society has become overly focused on constantly smelling like chemical fragrances. Don't let slick Madison Avenue ads impair your health. Of course, there are times when it's important to smell fresh and healthy deodorants are necessary. Whenever possible, though, let your sweat glands do what they were designed to do.

Deep Breathing

Breathing deeply on a regular basis is another important eliminative route. Benefits include releasing gaseous wastes and taking in lots of oxygen so vital for health. You can achieve deep breathing with exercise, singing, chanting, and romantic activities.

Other ways to breathe deeply include:

- *Cleansing breaths: take a slow deep breath in, hold to the count of four, and exhale slowly. Do 10 repetitions three times a day.*
- *Yoga breathing techniques called pranayama*
- *Holistic Breathing as discussed in the Awareness chapter*
- *Diaphragmatic breathing is done with less force, but longer than bellows breathing. This technique involves gently relaxing the abdominal muscles and letting them bulge out as you breathe in. As you breathe out, gently pull your stomach muscles in and up to assist complete exhalation. Use this way of breathing all the time, especially during meditation and other relaxation techniques*

- *Some people cannot breathe normally because of chronic sinus drainage. Sinus rinse kits, by NeilMed, for example, remove mucous and kill excess microorganisms that can cause chronic sinus conditions. Use this during allergy season, especially after exposure to grass cuttings, smoke, dust, and other fine particles.*
- *Sinus Relief™ and Super Neti Juice™ products by Natures Rite™ kill excess microorganisms in the sinuses.*

Blood Filtration

The liver, kidneys and spleen filter impurities from the blood. This information could save your life or that of a loved one like it did David.

David was a trim patient in his late fifties who took great care of himself, but developed chronic kidney failure with high blood pressure, swelling of the extremities, difficulty urinating, and extreme fatigue. His medical doctors had no idea why these problems started. They wanted him to start dialysis and warned about the likely occurrence of stroke and heart disease. Not a hopeful prognosis.

David heard about the power of natural healing methods and came to my office. I, too, was puzzled about a chronic disease in an otherwise very healthy appearing man until I read his history. He had worked in an aluminum plant for 30 years and was exposed to caustic chemicals and heavy metals dust. Mystery solved.

His kidneys showed an overload of—you guessed it—chemicals and heavy metals. Within a few months of helping his body remove the toxins, David was feeling better, urinating well, and his lower extremity swelling is down.

An easy and simple exercise that brings energy and percussion to these filtration organs. Here are the steps:

- *Sit up straight and raise your hands toward the ceiling with palms upward.*
- *Visualize 'sky chi' or energy from the universe filling your palms.*

- *Bring your elbows downward and firmly thump the front sides of your lower rib cage with the insides of your upper arms. This stimulates the liver and spleen.*
- *Repeat while striking the back sides of your rib cage to percuss the kidneys.*
- *Repeat 10 times over each area.*
- *Inhale while reaching toward the sky. Exhale while thumping over the organs.*

Steps to minimize the toxic load on these organs and assist optimal functioning include:

1. *Enjoy the real food way of eating and especially avoid trans fats*
2. *Drink alcohol very minimally if you choose to do so at all*
3. *Use a detox program such as the* ***Standard Process Purification Program*** *two to four times per year or as directed by your holistic health practitioner*
4. *Drink lots of pure water*
5. *Avoid or minimize prescription drugs that have harmful side effects to these organs. Especially beware if your medical doctor wants periodic liver and kidney tests after prescribing a drug.*
6. *Tone and massage these organs via yoga postures, an inversion table, visceral manipulations, or internal massage techniques*
7. *Attend to the other four eliminative routes*
8. *Use whole food nutritional products if necessary to help these filtering organs function optimally*

Secondary Eliminative Routes

If the five primary eliminative mechanisms are insufficient to remove wastes, *secondary eliminative processes* may occur. These are like internal spring cleanings that remove accumulated wastes and toxins.

For those not familiar with natural hygiene principles, a list of these backup cleansing mechanisms will look like a list of symptoms or diseases. They include:

1. *Sinus drainage*
2. *Sneezing*
3. *Coughing*
4. *Excessively heavy or prolonged menstrual periods*
5. *Boils, pimples, and skin rashes*
6. *Diarrhea*
7. *Heavy or overly smelly sweat*
8. *Vaginal discharge*
9. *Drainage from the eyes and ears*

While there other possible causes for these nine, they can simply be *cleansing crises symptoms* as the body resorts to extreme measures to remove waste products. These symptoms can often be prevented or reversed by improving the five primary ways of eliminating wastes. Secondary eliminative routes serve a valuable function in helping people heal themselves of serious illnesses. Here are two examples.

For over a year, Cathy had a steadily worsening trembling of her arms and hands. Psoriasis developed on her arms and she felt anxious and shaky inside. Worst of all, she thought she was losing her mind. An owner of a small business, she had been yelling at her customers for no reason at all and couldn't handle any stress.

Her *wake-up call* occurred when she was driving down a country road and a car full of teenagers passed her while honking and making obscene gestures. She went into a rage and followed them at high speed.

"My plan," she said, "was to run them off the road—you know, the way you see in the movies." Then she came to her senses and thought, "What am I doing?"

My evaluation showed excess chemicals and toxic metals affecting her brain. That made sense since her business exposed her to both of those daily. Within a week of starting the program, she developed large boils under both armpits that drained yellow-whitish pus. After a few weeks, the boils starting clearing up and so did Cathy's symptoms. Several years later, she only needs a maintenance checkup every three months and we celebrate her feeling great with no symptoms at all.

In retrospect, her symptoms made perfect sense. The psoriasis was nature's attempt to remove the toxins through the skin. Her neuromuscular and mental symptoms were the result of imbalance and stress in the brain.

Another patient I'll call Betty felt fine, but wanted to do the nutrition-based healing program to stay that way. Twenty years before, Betty had a benign lump removed from her left breast. Soon after that, she noticed fatty moles appearing on the left side of her chest and abdomen. A few weeks into the nutritional program, several of the moles split open and a clear fluid drained out. The fluid was so caustic that it severely burned her skin but Betty didn't care. "Whatever is draining," she said, "I'd rather have it out of me than in me!" Within a few weeks, the drainage stopped.

My theory is that her body developed the breast lump twenty years before in an attempt to wall off toxins. *The body is very intelligent and never does anything without a reason.* After the tumor was removed, her body resorted to storing the chemicals and heavy metals in fat much like radioactive wastes are stored in salt mines. Perhaps the detoxification program allowed her body to remove these substances so they didn't slowly leach into her system.

Healthy elimination can also decrease the frequency and severity of minor illnesses like a cold or flu. Our patients regularly remark that they are the only ones in their home or office who don't get sick when an illness is going around.

Microorganisms and Parasites

Microscopic bacteria, viruses, and yeast/fungus live inside the human body as do unicellular to large parasites. Collectively, they are potential *immune challenges.*

In a healthy person, good microorganisms—primarily bacteria and yeast called normal flora —are in a state of balance with 'bad' or more pathogenic strains. Three factors determine whether your body becomes overwhelmed by immune challenges:

1. *The number of microorganisms*
2. *Their virulence or strength*
3. *Your body's resistance*

Microorganisms vary in their infection causing potentials. For example, lactobacillus is a useful strain in yogurt while streptococcus is quite infectious. However, many natural health experts say that even pathogenic microorganisms are *helpful* in limited numbers.

These "bad guys" play a role in digesting dead matter—old cells, mucous, and other microorganisms. Bacteria, viruses, fungus/yeast, parasites, maggots, flies, buzzards, and possums are *scavengers.* They are one of nature's ways of disposing of dead and decaying material.

Regarding *host resistance,* French physiologist Claude Bernard said illnesses constantly hover above, but do not set in unless the terrain is ready to receive them. The body hosts many microorganisms, but if you are healthy and strong, you rarely become ill. An *internally clean* body won't support large numbers of harmful microorganisms.

Healthy people rarely get sick. Unhealthy ones with low immunity often catch illnesses. If *the number* of virulent microorganisms were the most important factor, health care providers would be ill all the time since they're often exposed to patients who have lots of germs. The most crucial factors in avoiding infections are:

1. *Increase your resistance and stay vibrantly healthy*
2. *Assist your body in controlling the numbers of immune challenges*

Regarding #1, this book outlines seven keys to getting and staying optimally well. For #2, nutrition-based healing methods help boost your body's immune system and control overgrowth of microorganisms.

Whenever possible, *assist* Mother Nature's attempts to heal and cleanse:

- *Minimize use of antibiotics because they kill normal flora and upset the balance of 'good' and 'bad' microorganisms.*
- *If you must use antibiotics, also take whole food supplements to reestablish populations of good bacteria and yeast.*
- *Enjoy the real food way of eating. Strictly limit your intake of sugar, junk food, and excess carbs. Microorganisms feed on sugar and over populate if you eat too much.*
- *Ensure normal elimination of wastes with bowel movements, urination, deep breathing and sweating.*
- *Remember the healing power of extra rest and sleep.*
- *Some sneezing and coughing eliminate wastes from the sinuses and lungs so don't suppress these cleansing routes. However, if severe coughing stops you from resting, use natural preparations such as* ***B & T cough syrup*** *and* ***Olba's throat lozenges****.*
- *Diarrhea and vomiting clear out the gastrointestinal tract and stomach. Within reason, let these processes run their course. Ditto for skin rashes, boils, pimples and other secondary eliminative routes to remove wastes.*
- *Whenever possible, don't suppress a fever by using tepid baths or drugs. For children, a fever up to 104 degrees Fahrenheit orally is good because it kills pathogenic microorganisms. Always consult your doctor since properly managing a fever depends on the patient's age, health status, signs and symptoms, etc.*
- *Avoid exposure to people who are ill with an active infection.*
- *Avoid flu and other vaccinations that inject live or weakened bacteria or viruses into your body and past the normal immune defenses. As discussed in the* ***Natural Care*** *chapter, vaccinations have questionable effectiveness, clear short-term dangers, and unknown long-term health consequences.*

- *Avoid over-the-counter and prescription drugs that decrease stomach acid levels. Sufficient gastric juice acidity is needed to kill pathogenic bacteria that enter via the stomach. Normal stomach function is also crucial for mineral absorption needed by the immune system.*
- *Follow the **Immunity Enhancement Program** (see appendix H) at the first sign of a cold, flu or other infection.*

Excess Chemicals

Chemicals are all around you – in food, air, water, body care products, home and laundry cleaning products, etc.

The Environmental Protection Agency estimates that the average American comes into contact with over 2000 chemicals a day. The U.S. allows over 14,000 chemicals to be in our food supply. Newborn babies have been found with hundreds of chemicals in their blood.

Until big businesses put health concerns before profit, chemicals will abound. A popular phrase in the 1960's was: "Better living through chemistry." Fifty years later, we're seeing the negative impacts on our health.

Excessive chemicals are harmful, especially in the amounts present today. Your body can tolerate some unnaturally occurring chemicals, but not in the current excessive forms and amounts. Chemicals particularly affect the brain and hormonal glands, thus causing common physical and mental symptoms.

Sherry Rogers MD, author of *Detoxify or Die,* states that chemicals and heavy metals are also often a core cause of neuromuscular diseases such as Parkinson's, Lou Gehrig's, Multiple Sclerosis, and other afflictions involving tremors.

Those whose jobs involve *chemical exposure* are especially vulnerable to developing these types of disorders. Linda, a forty-five-year-old who had worked around chemicals for 20 years, developed tremors of the hands and an autoimmune disorder.

She said several coworkers in their mid-thirties also had tremors of the face and hands. Her symptoms cleared up nicely when we helped her body remove the over-accumulation of chemicals.

Excess chemicals need to be dealt with for ourselves, our children and our children's children. Otherwise, more and more people will likely face major illness and mental imbalances. If traditional medical care is sought, the treatment will usually be more chemicals in the form of prescription drugs.

When making important decisions centuries ago, Native Americans considered the impact on *seven generations ahead.* Unfortunately, many of today's decisions are based on profit while future health impacts are ignored.

Everyday in my practice, I see heart-wrenching examples of people whose lives are impaired or ruined by excess chemicals. We have seen a number of teenagers who suffer with ten or more serious symptoms such as depression, anxiety, difficulty concentrating, fatigue, insomnia, morbid fears, nightmares, etc.

Since chemicals are inescapable and harmful, you are wise to minimize your exposure and regularly remove them from your body.

Chemical categories and their most common sources include:

Body Care Products: nonnatural brands of facial creams, artificial nails, lotions, oils, shampoo and conditioner, soap, powders, breath freshener, makeup, hair gels/ coloring, mouthwash, cologne, shaving cream, toothpaste, baby wipes and diapers

Home Cleaners: any commercial home cleaners that contain chemicals. Instead, use natural products containing baking soda, white vinegar, lemon, borax, castile soap, salt, and essential oils for fragrance.

Food Dyes: in processed and packages foods with food coloring added

Food Preservatives: in packaged and processed foods and some salad bars

Formaldehyde: permanent press and other treated fabrics, cosmetics and toiletries, household cleaners, paper products, building materials, medications, paint and stripping agents, cigarettes, smoke from burning wood, etc.

Herbicides: non-organic foods and unfiltered water

Medications: prescription drugs

Acetate/Acetone: paint, varnish, nail polish and remover, paint thinners and removers, cosmetics, artificial flavors, adhesives

Hydrocarbons: exhaust from gas or diesel engines, and natural gas

Petrosolvents: paints, varnishes, glues, adhesives, aerosol sprays, ink, permanent markers, solvents such as benzene and carbon tetrachloride

Pesticides: chemical products used to control bugs and plants

Plastic: plastic wrap, plastic water bottles, food packaging

In addition to minimizing exposure to the sources above, what else can you do?

- *Use **naturally based body care products** whenever possible. Avoid ones that contain chemical fragrances, colors, and preservatives.*
- *When you are around new furniture, building materials or car, thoroughly ventilate the area, especially in bedrooms.*
- *Filter water used for drinking and bathing to avoid common chemicals in tap water. Don't flush harmful chemicals such as unused prescription drugs and paint down the toilet or sink.*

- *Eat real food from local organic sources to avoid dyes, food preservatives, and chemicals from containers. Avoid foods that have been treated with herbicides and pesticides. Don't eat meat, eggs or dairy products that have been raised with growth hormones, antibiotics, and chemicals.*
- *Use naturally-based house cleaning and pesticide products.*
- *Read labels: it's not a good sign if a food, body care, or housecleaning product contains lots of long chemical-sounding words that you can't pronounce.*
- *Contact your legislators and urge their action to protect people, animals and the environment from chemical products and wastes.*
- *Use healthy elimination and detox measures described earlier in this chapter.*
- *Lose weight if needed since chemicals and heavy metals can store in fat*
- *Use a detox program such as the* ***Standard Process Purification Program*** *two to four times a year to assist internal cleansing of the bowels, kidneys, lungs, blood, lymphatics and skin.*
- *Use a nutrition-based healing program to detect excess chemicals and determine what approach is best to remove them.*

Hiding your head in the sand isn't going to make this one go away. There are many advantages of 21st century living, but chemical toxicity must be addressed or more people, especially children will suffer.

Toxic Metals

Toxic or heavy metals – for example, mercury, aluminum, arsenic, plutonium and lead – can cause serious illness. Others, such as iron, copper, manganese and zinc, are needed in small amounts but cause damage at excessive levels.

Pollution of air, food and water has increased the amount of certain metals that pose health risks for humans and animals. Other heavy metals are *purposely added* to products. Example include aluminum in antiperspirant deodorants, or mercury in vaccinations, dental fillings and processed foods. These are present in small amounts that over time can accumulate and contribute to disease.

Certain individuals are *more sensitive* to these metals and are like a canary in a coal mine—a first line alert of coming danger to others.

Many doctors and health scientists point to the serious health problems these days and consider heavy metal toxicity to be a core cause. For example, consider the large Alzheimer's treatment centers in existence these days. When I was young, I was around many older people in our family, neighborhood and church. None of them had dementia, senility, Alzheimer's or whatever label is used to describe the alarming incidence of memory loss and mental confusion.

In my holistic health care centers, we have treated a number of people *in their thirties and forties* who report significant problems with memory and concentration.

Why are so many children suffering with mental symptoms such as hyperactivity, depression, anxiety and behavior problems? Same question with adults who have facial or hand tremors before middle age. What is going on? Many experts are pointing to the increase in toxic metals and urging people to face this problem now.

Toxic metals and their common sources include:

Aluminum: cookware, packaged foods, antacids, antiperspirants, baking soda, aluminum cans, kitchen utensils, paints, dental composites, toothpaste

Antimony: flame-retardant clothing and furniture, medicines, pigments

Arsenic: poisons, pigments, dyes, wood preservative, insecticide, wine, well water, coal burning, shellfish, treated lumber

Barium: diagnostic tests, drinking water, bleaches, dyes, fireworks, ceramics

Beryllium: exposure at nuclear and aerospace industries, refining and melting of beryllium-containing alloys, manufacturing of electronic devices

Bromine: agriculture chemicals, flame-retardants, contaminated drinking water and food sources, spas, swimming pools

Cadmium: fertilizers, cigarettes, water from galvanized pipes, shellfish, industrial fumes, paint, air pollution, auto exhaust

Calcium: poor quality sources of calcium, excess dairy products

Chromium: cheap chromium-coated stainless steel kitchen utensils corroded by acidic foods, dyes, pigments, air pollution, dental crowns

Copper: poor quality mineral supplements, copper plumbing, cook ware, dental materials, pesticides, jewelry, IUDs, birth control pills

Fluorine: fluoride containing toothpaste and mouthwash, fluoridated water

Gold/Silver: cheap jewelry, dental fillings, injections for arthritis

Iodine: excess supplements and iodized salt, topical iodine solution

Iron: paints, dyes, poor quality mineral supplements, enriched wheat flour, pollution, occupational exposure, tobacco

Lead: paint, car exhaust, occupational exposure, plumbing, canned food, hair dye

Magnesium: poor quality mineral supplements, antacids, laxatives

Manganese: well water, ceramics, dyes, medicines, job exposure

Mercury: processed foods, dental fillings, seafood, vaccinations, water

Nickel: auto exhaust, cigarettes, dental crowns, occupational exposure

Radioactive Metals: contaminated food, air and water; nuclear plants

Tin: canned foods, paints, pesticides, contaminated water, job exposure

Titanium: paints, medications, orthopedic/dental implants, job exposure

Zinc: poor quality mineral supplements, exposure to smelters, metal cans

What *action steps* can you take so toxic metals don't hurt you and your loved ones?

1. *Prevention of further heavy metals listed above*
2. *Removal of toxic metals already in the body.*

Prevention involves *avoiding further exposure* to the above sources as much as possible. Suggestions for doing this include:

- *Avoid processed foods, especially those containing high fructose corn syrup, as much as possible since they can contain small amounts of mercury as a preservative*
- *Use deodorants with natural ingredients, not aluminum*
- *Don't use canned foods to prevent intake of lead, aluminum, tin and other metals*
- *Avoid medical drugs as much as possible since they may contain heavy metals; this is especially critical for vaccinations that can contain mercury in the form of thimerosal*
- *Use a mercury-free dentist for your dental fillings*
- *Filter drinking water with a dual carbon filter, and bathing water with a wholehouse filter*

- *Avoid over-the-counter medications, for example, antacids that contain toxic metals*
- *Use skin care products that only contain natural ingredients*

You get the idea: look at the list of common sources and eliminate them as much as possible. Be sure to tell your family and friends about the dangers of heavy metals so they can avoid them, too.

Finally, be sure to contact your legislators and urge their action to protect people, animals and the environment from toxic metals.

For *treatment,* use the same healing programs as with chemicals.

Scars

Have you ever heard the phrase, "She was scarred for life"? It usually refers to *emotional scars* and the lasting impact those can have on a person. *Physical scars* can also negatively impact your health.

Scars are defined as anything that breaks the surface of the skin: surgery, cuts, injuries, animal or insect bites, injections, IV sites/ports, burns, stretch marks, body piercings and tattoos. Areas with old or active acne, boils, rashes or open sores can also act as scars. Scars are sometimes a significant cause of severe health problems.

Mary had been perfectly healthy until age thirty-five and the birth of her third child. Then it was all downhill. At age fifty-five, despite the best of conventional and natural health care, she was a cardiac invalid who was completely bed-ridden and looked seventy-five.

Finally, someone told her about nutrition-based healing approaches and she was evaluated. Her doctor found that scars from an episiotomy and perineal tear during childbirth were negatively affecting the energy flows to her cardiovascular system. After treating the scars at home for several weeks, she began improving. One year later, she was totally healthy and looked and acted much younger than her age.

How can scars negatively impact your health? One part of your nervous system, the *sympathetic* nervous system (SNS), regulates active functions. The parasympathetic nervous system (PSNS) controls relaxation functions: sleep, optimal digestion and sexual arousal. The SNS and PSNS ideally predominate when appropriate.

SNS fibers terminate or end on the surface of the skin. These fibers are so vast in number that an outline of your form would still be visible if everything else about you were dissolved.

Normally, SNS fibers relay information in the form of nerve impulses to and from the brain. However, scars can disrupt normal communication and energy transmission. Instead of flowing smoothly, energy can build up at the scar site and discharge in an unbalanced manner. Over time, organ dysfunction and associated symptoms can result.

I've seen scar treatment help numerous people who suffered from chronic symptoms. These patients had tried everything else and were motivated to try something new.

Debra developed childhood diabetes within months of a serious electrical shock that left a large scar on her hand. Dustin had heart symptoms that responded wonderfully when his scars and other stressors were treated. Terry had depression and anxiety due to, in part, her scars short-circuiting normal nervous system function.

Scars along the *midline of the body* – for example, from a hysterectomy, episiotomy, C-section, circumcision, vasectomy, or open-heart surgery – are especially problematic. These scars cross major meridian or energy pathways that are recognized by doctors of oriental medicine and acupuncturists. When the energy flow is disrupted, associated organs can suffer.

What can you do to prevent scars from affecting your health and energy? First, *avoid creating new scars* as much as possible. Avoid getting tattoos since they act as scars and inject heavy metals into the body. If you must pierce your body with jewelry, limit it to one per ear in the usual spot and with only small earrings.

Unless it's an emergency situation, have surgical procedures only as a last resort and after trying natural healing methods. Prevent animal and insect bites and cuts as much as possible. Not all scars cause health problems, but it's wise to minimize them. Scars that are stressing your body can be identified with a nutrition-based healing method such as Nutrition Response Testing.

If you already have scars, firmly rub fresh wheat germ or sesame seed oil over the scars for three minutes daily for sixty days. This helps about 50 percent of active cases. Low intensity laser light therapy usually handles the other 50 percent.

EMF: Electromagnetic Fields

A growing body of research indicates serious potential health dangers of excess *electromagnetic fields* (EMF.) Scientists have known about these dangers for decades after investigating sick and dying cattle that lived under high energy power lines.

Since then, reputable research and epidemiological studies have been done and the verdict is clear. However, as with cigarettes, most doctors and the public are slow to realize the negative impact. Meanwhile, people are suffering and dying needlessly and prematurely from the harmful effects of EMF.

Here's a statistic that might get your attention. Currently, people are exposed to 100 million times the EMF that their grandparents were and the amount is increasing each year. Many of the body's physiological processes – from sleep cycles to immune strength to DNA genetic expression – can be influenced by excess EMF.

Natural EMF is produced by the earth and every cell of the human body. This low intensity EMF is natural and conducive to good health.

The problem arises with *artificial EMF.* Every electronic device, from hairdryers to cell phones to cell towers, produce high intensity electromagnetic energy that interferes with the body's natural energy field.

The *electrical field portion* emanates from the device even when it is turned off, but it is easy to block with metal. However, the magnetic field is only released when the device is turned on, but is impossible to block—even with metal or concrete.

Both types of fields are completely silent and invisible. How do you know if there is excess EMF around you? If your area receives cell phone service or electric power, it is.

The *National Institute of Environmental Health Sciences,* after a review of over 2000 scientific studies on EMF, concluded that it should be regarded as possibly carcinogenic. These studies show that excessive EMF weakens the body's resistance to microorganisms and increases the risk of cancer.

The list of conditions associated with excess EMF includes: memory loss, birth defects, impaired immunity, mood swings, depression, violent behavior, chronic stress and suicide.

What can you do about it? *Minimizing exposure* is one key because, in most civilized areas, escaping it completely is not possible. Live and work as far away as possible from cellular towers and large electrical transmitting and power stations. Avoid using microwaves and electric blankets. Don't keep your cell phone on your body or bedside table. During longer cell phone conversations, use light headphones or ear buds with a long cord with the cell phone distant from your body.

Especially avoid being near sources of *dirty electricity* that you don't really need: dimmer switches, power saving fluorescent light bulbs, halogen lamps, and older fluorescent lighting systems.

Wireless routers, computers, copy machines, television sets, and cell phone chargers are used by most people. One solution is to keep them unplugged except when in use and stay as far away from them as possible when they are.

Another key to minimizing EMF is to keep a simple protective device on or near your body. I use the *Vitaplex* and *SafeSpace Protection* devices from ***SafeSpaceProtection.com***. I recommend these for everyone, especially those who test positive for EMF with nutrition-based healing approaches.

For more information about this important topic, read *Dirty Electricity: Electrification and the Diseases of Civilization* by Samuel Milham MD, MPH; *Electromagnetic Fields: A Consumer's Guide to the Issues and How to Protect Ourselves* by B. Blake Levitt; and *Cross Currents* by Robert O. Becker MD.

Visit the website of Joseph Mercola DO (***Mercola.com***) to learn more the dangers of EMF and what you can do about it. The site ***SafeSpaceProtection.com*** is another good source of information and to protect you and your loved ones from the dangers of EMF.

Infrared Sauna

Infrared sauna uses *radiant heat* and is an excellent way to internally cleanse your body. Infrared energy is the portion of the electromagnetic spectrum that provides the sun's warmth and is the type of heat that is produced by the body's cells. Infrared heat is so safe that it is used in incubators to warm newborn babies. Research in Japan and Sweden indicates that infrared is a safe form of electromagnetic exposure.

Sauna usage dates back at least several thousand years B.C. and has been used by cultures as diverse as Native Americans, Scandinavians and Tibetans for its holistic benefits. Traditionally, saunas were very hot with temperatures of 180 to 235 degrees Fahrenheit. *Infrared sauna,* however, is therapeutic at only 110 to 130 degrees.

Despite being much cooler, infrared saunas allow the body to sweat more than high temperature units. The cooler temperature makes it more comfortable, easier to breathe, and eliminates cardiovascular risks associated with increased heat.

Infrared rays have been researched extensively, particularly in Japan and Europe. Health benefits include:

1. *Detoxification of heavy metals, chemicals and other wastes*
2. *Cardiovascular conditioning due to increase in heart volume and rate*
3. *Weight loss: 30 minutes in a sauna can burn 900 or more calories*
4. *Musculoskeletal benefits for arthritis, muscle spasm, pain, adhesions, joint stiffness, bursitis, strains, and sprains*
5. *Improved skin conditions such as acne, psoriasis, and eczema*
6. *Increased blood flow throughout the body*
7. *Deep relaxation of muscles with stress reducing effects*

Contra-indications for infrared sauna include: pregnancy, injuries less than 48 hours old, and hemophilia or any predisposition to excess bleeding. In addition, check with your physician if you have any disease; are on medications; have metal pins, rods, artificial joints, or surgical implants; have silicone implants of any type.

Leonard Smith MD and Brenda Watson, authors of *The Detox Strategy,* recommend the TheraSauna company (***TheraSauna.com***). We have a product from that company in our home. My office can serve as a distributor. You can check the specifications of their products to evaluate the quality of other infrared sauna systems.

Practicing Environmental Awareness

Caring for the environment is another key to inner cleanliness since it ensures healthier food, air, and water. An ancient Navajo prophecy stated: "If we dare to pollute the land and water, we will all suffer the consequences." That is already occurring.

This planet is living and responsive, not a huge inert sphere that can be endlessly abused without negative repercussions. We can no longer tolerate thoughtless or profit driven pollution and abuse of our planet.

On a positive note, the *I Ching* encourages: "What has been spoiled through man's fault can be made good again through man's work." Here are nine basic recommendations from ***ClimateCrisis.net***:

1. *Walk, bike, carpool, or take mass transit more often*
2. *Recycle and reuse*
3. *Keep your car tires fully inflated*
4. *Use less hot water: use a low flow shower head and wash clothes in cold or warm water*
5. *Avoid products with lots of packaging*
6. *Adjust your thermostat down 2 degrees in the winter and up 2 degrees in the summer*
7. *Plant one or more trees and support wildlife conservation areas*
8. *Learn more and get active to be part of the solution*

The ecosphere has corrective measures that can help remedy problems if given a chance. So it's not hopeless; our immediate and unified responses can help. Technology, people, and nature *can work together responsibly* without doing each other harm. The next step beyond high tech can be clean tech as new technologies become more sophisticated and environmentally sensitive.

Learn and follow recommendations for a healthy environment. Each of us can make a difference. As Edmund Burke said, "Nobody made a greater mistake than he who did nothing because he could only do a little." Resources for further information include:

- ***50 Simple Things You Can Do to Save The Earth*** *by the EarthWorks Group*
- ***How to Make the World a Better Place*** *by Jeffrey Hollender*
- ***Empty Harvest*** *by Mark Anderson and Bernard Jensen DC*
- *The book and Academy Award-winning documentaries* ***An Inconvenient Truth*** *and* ***An Inconvenient Sequel: Truth to Power*** *by former senator and vice-president Al Gore*

No Tobacco Products

Avoiding smoking, second hand smoke and smokeless tobacco is of utmost importance for inner cleanliness and *radiant wellness.*

Nearly 500,000 Americans die each year from tobacco related diseases. While a respiratory therapist, I saw thousands of people suffer needlessly and die prematurely because of cigarettes. The end stages of chronic lung disease are a living hell.

Mary was crying as she sat up late at night shortly before she died, trying to get a breath. She looked at me with eyes already glimpsing the next realm and implored me to warn others: "We didn't know how dangerous cigarettes were when I started smoking. Please tell others so they won't have to go through what I have." Many patients have similarly begged me to warn others about the dangers of smoking before it's too late.

So I'm warning.

Avoiding tobacco products is just common sense – much like fastening your seat belt, paying attention while driving, not drinking your self stupid, and avoiding drugs. Many common illnesses and deaths could be prevented if people would just treat themselves and others with more love and respect.

You can experience what it's like to suffer from a terminal lung disease. Cover your mouth with one hand and pinch off your nostrils with the other hand. Now breathe for a couple of minutes. You can't, right? What a relief to be able to remove your hands and breathe. But there is no relief for severe lung disease patients except death.

It's virtually impossible to enjoy radiant wellness if you smoke much. I've heard about chronic smokers who live long lives and have seen some of them. Their skin looks like a prune and their lungs gurgle when they talk and laugh in between painful coughing jags.

Cigarette smoke is almost 200 degrees Fahrenheit, nearly the temperature at which water boils. No wonder the mouth, sinuses, throat, and lungs undergo degenerative changes, cellular mutation and cancer. Health care and lost work time costs due to smoking are over $300 billion each year in the U.S. alone. The cost in human suffering and shortened lives cannot be measured.

Nicotine is as physically addictive as heroin so compassion and professional help are needed. I realized how addictive smoking is when I was working in hospitals as a respiratory therapist. Some of the patients had *tracheotomies,* an opening in their throats that they breathed through. While checking patients on oxygen during late night rounds, I found a patient smoking a cigarette through his tracheotomy! This thirty-eight-year-old man died within the week.

Various smoking cessation programs are available at little or no cost. Addressing nutritional deficiencies is another key to stopping. For any program to succeed over time, a person has to really want to quit. Hypnotherapy, acupuncture, and herbal formulas can help. Nicotine substitutes and medications are needed by some people.

You can quit if you really want to. A big key to successfully quitting is having sufficient motivation. Over the years, I've heard many patients *say* they'll stop some day. Or they *try* to quit but fail time after time. When they're diagnosed with lung cancer or serious heart disease, however, they quit instantly. Why wait until it's too late?

The first three to five days without cigarettes or other tobacco products are the worst *so just get it over with.* Assemble your health care team to help you live without this fatal chemical crutch.

Strategies for becoming free from tobacco addiction include:

- *Mild to moderate aerobic exercise five days a week*
- *Take 10 slow deep breaths every time you crave a cigarette*
- *Pray for inner strength and spiritual guidance*
- *Relax by meditating, spending time in nature, and hobbies*
- *Use whole food supplements and the real food way of eating to become optimally well and increase your energy naturally*

- *Use herbal formulas to detox and lessen nicotine cravings*
- *Enlist friends to support your new tobacco-free lifestyle*
- *Remove all cigarettes and ashtrays from your home*
- *Have oral alternatives handy: gum, toothpicks, mints, vegetable slices, or gum with healthy sweeteners*
- *Create different patterns not associated with smoking. For example, if you always smoked after a meal, get away from the table and engage in some other activity after eating*
- *Get your teeth whitened to remove tobacco stains*
- *Celebrate by going somewhere that is smoke-free*

Use Alcohol Minimally or Not At All

In our society, alcohol is the most widely accepted way to change ones state of consciousness. People enjoy looking at life from a different perspective and alcohol allows that. It's fun to feel a little giddy, laugh, and be relaxed. Those are good things.

Some studies even suggest that very moderate drinking—one or two glasses of wine a day, for example—provides minor health benefits. However, there are other ways to achieve those benefits. Other studies say that any benefits are outweighed by negative factors and the potential for addiction.

About 10 percent of our population become alcoholics who, by genetic predisposition or acquired addiction or both, cannot drink moderately. Unfortunately, most people don't know they are an alcoholic until it is too late.

Signs and symptoms for being at risk for alcoholism include: morning drinking, blackouts, regrettable actions while intoxicated, trouble stopping, five or more drinks per day, friends and family becoming concerned, interference with your job, driving under the influence, and a family history of alcoholism.

If you choose to use alcohol, wait until legal age and *don't drive while drinking!* At least 50 percent of America's fatal traffic accidents involve alcohol.

I understand the severity of the problem. My family has a multigenerational history of alcoholism, depression and blood sugar handling disorders. Alcohol provides instant jet fuel that temporarily raises blood sugar levels and causes euphoria.

In addition to Alcoholics Anonymous and medical supervision, I recommend using the seven keys to radiant wellness. Natural health practices can also be a potent aid in preventing and treating alcoholism.

If you're *not* an alcoholic, you can enjoy moderate and responsible drinking. However, in certain individuals over time, *even moderate* alcohol intake can cause impaired liver function, brain cell damage, gastric and esophageal irritation, and yeast infections.

Just recently, a new patient told me about his indigestion symptoms. At age 26, he's been on medication for gastroesophageal reflux disease (GERD) for several years. He was wearing a T-shirt and hat with beer logos so I took a stab in the dark and asked about his drinking habits. He admitted to drinking five beers, five days a week for several years so it's probably more than that. You can imagine what decades of alcohol abuse can bring.

One final note. Those who take great care of themselves and receive natural health care may feel crummy after drinking even moderate amounts of alcohol, especially hard liquor, beer, or wine with preservatives. Good wine or beer *without chemical additives* seems to work best for those who can and want to drink in moderation.

Many years ago, my brother-in-law talked me into celebrating his 50th birthday by drinking beer with him. I hadn't drunk any alcohol for many years, but three cold ones went down pretty smoothly. I felt a little dizzy two hours later so I went to bed. In the middle of the night, I woke up and felt very dizzy. A hangover was my constant companion for the next two days with headache, malaise, and lack of mental clarity. Needless to say, it wasn't worth the buzz.

When you're radiantly well, drinking bacteria urine – which is what alcohol is – constitutes an inferior high.

Avoid Illegal Drugs

Here's another disastrous wrong turn that creates inner toxicity and much worse. Drug use has created vast suffering for many people. Everyone wants to feel good and, granted, drugs can provide a fleeting high but at such a cost. Fortunately, there are better *natural ways* to relax and feel great without using drugs.

In my youth, I tried various ways of altering my consciousness. Fortunately, however, I soon saw that no matter how 'high' I got, I always came down. And there was that silly little matter of feeling hung over and wiped out for a day or two. I noticed that pot heads and heavy drinkers started to look and act brain damaged. I decided that there had to be a better way.

There is.

Some people consider *recreational* use of drugs to be harmless and cool. Webster defines recreational as "creating anew or refreshing in body or mind" but there is nothing renewing or refreshing about drug use. I've observed the tragic downsides firsthand and the lessons are clear: it's better to never start. Some people who plan to try it just once become psychologically and physiologically addicted or damaged.

Drug use increases the incidence of robberies, accidents, murder, suicide, domestic violence, and child abuse. The cost in lost potential due to lowered standards and poor life decisions cannot be estimated. My recommendation is to steer clear of all illegal drugs since they can cause significant personal, family, and societal problems.

Pressures to experiment with drugs can be powerful, especially during one's youth. However, drugs are illegal, can be dangerous, and can lead to unwise behaviors. No matter how finely tuned the dose or well designed the drug, you always come down. The chemicals in drugs are often cumulative and their long-term effects are unknown.

Even marijuana – considered a harmless and even beneficial herb by many – has 400 different chemicals in it. When smoked as a joint, the burning paper and pot combination releases over 2,000 chemicals. Some of these fat soluble chemicals accumulate in organs and can cause short and long-term impairments.

Many people enjoy – depending on the strain and amount used – varying degrees of relaxation/energy, mental clarity/comfortably numb, and almost always euphoria with marijuana. With legalization in a growing number of states, its use will probably increase. And, frankly, I usually would rather see my patients smoke a few tokes of vaporized good quality pot in the safety of their home than get drunk.

However, there are still potential risks, especially if a person drives while stoned. Using pot could lead to experimenting with other drugs since it clearly lowers inhibitions. And there's the chance of decreased motivation and psychological addiction. All things considered, I still recommend getting and staying high naturally.

Young people, please don't make the same mistakes that prior generations have with more dangerous drugs. Visit mental hospitals and chemical dependency units and see the potential results of drug abuse for yourself. During my pastoral counseling practicum at a psychiatric hospital, I met Jim, a sixteen-year-old boy who had taken PCP. Despite a year of treatment, Jim was a walking vegetable and will probably be in a mental institution for the rest of his life.

Haven't we individually and collectively suffered enough? Please focus on natural ways of looking, feeling and being your very best. By the way, some people use drugs because those sometimes provide a *glimpse* of inner peace and enlightenment. Why not pursue a natural path that helps you reach these sublime states and stay there most or all the time?

Decades of drug experimentation have left a clear conclusion: there is no safe, legal or effective way to stay high on drugs. God knows, enough people have tried and paid a tragic price for the experiment. Wise ones will learn from the experience of others and evolve toward better ways of feeling great.

The Bottom Line

The most important points in the *Inner Cleanse* chapter include:

1. *Properly eliminate wastes with bowel movements, urination, sweating and deep breathing*
2. *Reduce waste removal loads by eating chemical-free food and water*
3. *Assist waste removal with saunas, purification programs, and herbal cleanses*
4. *Minimize exposure to and remove toxic metals, excess chemicals, scars, and electromagnetic radiation*
5. *Practice environmental awareness so we and future generations have clean air, water, and soil*
6. *Don't smoke or use smokeless tobacco*
7. *Use alcohol minimally or not at all*
8. *Avoid illegal drugs, ideally even 'recreational' ones like pot*

Action Steps for Inner Cleansing Your Body

List two action steps you commit to starting within 30 days:

1. ______________________________
2. ______________________________

List two action steps you commit to starting within 60 days:

1. ______________________________
2. ______________________________

List two action steps you commit to starting within 90 days:

1. ______________________________
2. ______________________________

R
A
D
I
Awareness
N
T

Key #5
Awareness

"As a man thinketh in his heart, so shall he be..." —Jesus

"Our life is what our thoughts make it." —Marcus Aurelius

If all the existing *information and energy* – what life is ultimately comprised of – were the size of Mt. Everest, your five senses only can detect a portion the size of a golf ball. Seeing more of the bigger picture of life helps your life make more sense, especially when going through big changes and challenges. That's why it's so important to increase your awareness.

In the past, you likely looked at reality as though through a tiny pinhole in a wall. You only saw a minute fraction of the completeness of life, so you naturally assumed that's all there was. With that limited vision, you may have suffered with misunderstandings, for example:

- *death is the end of life*
- *you will never see your 'departed' loved ones again*
- *life is cruel, chaotic, and meaningless*
- *any Higher Power, if one really exists, is ignorant, uncaring, and impotent*

Fortunately, there is much more to life than meets the eye and none of those beliefs appear to be true.

Clear awareness is vital because, as the opening quotes indicate, your thoughts attract what comes into your life. Synonyms for *awareness* include: aliveness, attentiveness, consciousness, discernment, enlightenment, mindfulness, realization, and understanding. Are those some attributes you want more of in your life?

You have an inner wisdom that knows what to do and can make the best decisions to keep you healthy, happy and energetic. Being in touch with your innate intelligence is a major key to enjoying *radiant wellness.*

The goal of any wise physician is to improve a person's awareness. Then the patient *doesn't have to be told* how to eat, exercise, rest, and so on. The person's inner wisdom knows how to live. How often do you check in with your inner wisdom?

You've no doubt heard someone say, "He and I just aren't on the same wavelength!" You know how that feels and the problems it can create. My question to you is: are you on the same wavelength with yourself?

Increasing your awareness is a multifaceted endeavor so please be patient as I cover the bases. First and foremost, make improving your awareness a high priority. You've heard it said, "When you die, you can't take it with you." Your level of consciousness is one exception. Thus, wise people take time to cultivate clear mindfulness.

Perspective

Every day is a new opportunity for loving, service, adventure, growth and enjoyment. Viewing life with this perspective helps you appreciate every precious moment.

As you journey down life's path, focus on the bigger picture and look past trivial or temporary obstacles. Strive for an enlightened perspective like Winston Churchill who had inscribed on his tomb, "And this too shall pass."

Ancient Chinese and Egyptian symbols depicted *opportunity and crisis* as two sides of the same coin. Developing a positive perspective allows you to grow and learn from all life's experiences. The challenge is to *find the blessings* in each moment.

As Napoleon Hill, author of *Think and Grow Rich,* stated: "Every adversity, every failure and every heartache carries with it the seed of an equivalent or a greater benefit." There are good reasons for popular phrases such as: "There's a silver lining to every cloud; when one door closes, another opens; and always look for the blessings."

Remember, you always have the *power to choose* your outlook. It's the old partial glass of water question: it's half full to the optimist and half empty to the pessimist. *Focus on what you want,* not what you don't want, since you become what you most fervently think about.

How do you look at life? John Milton said, "The mind is its own place, and in itself, can make a Heaven of Hell, a Hell of Heaven." Which way you look at life literally creates the world you live in. A positive perspective is a powerful ally for every aspect of your life.

Keys to Increased Awareness

1. ***Create a pro and con list*** *whenever faced with difficult decisions. List the advantages and disadvantages of each decision and notice which list is longer. Prioritize the items and see which ones are most important to you. Viewing your options in black and white often clarifies decision-making.*
2. ***Future tripping,*** *a simple visualization technique, helps you through tough times. Imagine ahead 1, 5, 10, or more years and see yourself being successful and happy. Picture reaching your goals in spite of or even because of the difficulties you presently face. Remind yourself that most major stressors are time-limited so enjoy your visions of a brighter tomorrow.*
3. ***The 80/10/10 Rule*** *states that 100 percent success all the time is impossible. Unrealistically high expectations set you up for failure and self-criticism. Things will usually go smoothly 80 percent of the time and fairly well another 10%. The other 10% are events*

governed by Murphy's Law. So if you reach your goals 80% of the time with gusts of 90%, that's great. Whenever things get rough, mentally remind yourself 80/10/10.

4. ***Appreciate what you have** and give thanks for it. Happiness is being content with what you have and, at the same time, growing toward even greater heights. So, yes, set your goals and never stop improving, but remember that happiness lies in the journey and in reaching the destination.*

   Also, remember that the grass often seems greener on the other side of the fence. Some people waste their lives chasing the carrot dangling in front of them: a new car, bigger home, more attractive partner, and so on. They don't realize that lasting happiness does not come from ego boosts or material objects.

   None of this, by the way, is a justification for mediocrity or putting up with a chronically unhappy situation.

5. ***Count your blessings** rather than focusing on the negative. We all have so much to be thankful for. I learned this lesson at college when I was going bald. I envied a thick haired student who was walking on the other side of a short concrete wall. As he passed the wall, however, I saw that he had only one leg. It reminded me of the saying, "I complained about having no shoes until I met a man with no feet."*

6. ***Don't take life too seriously.** Humor and laughter are important for psychological and physical balance. Research shows an increased immune response, decreased anxiety, and reduced muscular tension with hearty laughter. Since prevention is the best approach, take time to regularly enjoy humor from comedians, children, everyday life, and televangelists.*

7. ***Motivational books and tapes** keep your heart and mind focused more positively. With a steady input of higher thought, you can look at the bright side more consistently. Enrich your life with the works of positive and enthusiastic individuals. By the way, the word enthusiasm comes from two root words meaning 'filled with God.'*

   Over the years, I've particularly benefited from inspirational teachings by Richard Bach, Wayne Dyer, Denis Waitley, Og Mandino, Richard Carlson, Stephen Covey, David Schwartz, Charles "Tremendous" Jones, Zig Ziglar and others.

8. ***Take it easy on the material things.*** *More is not always better. The stress in your life is directly proportional to the number of electronic and gasoline-powered objects you own. Keeping up with the Joneses can keep you overworked, stressed out, and broke. Slick advertisements by big businesses influence you to buy things that you don't need and you can't afford.*

9. ***Form a Master Mind group.*** *Find several people who want to improve their lives. Meet once or twice a month to discuss action plans for how to do that. Stay focused and positive; don't let it become a complaining session or social hour. Your Master Mind allies can provide valuable feedback, support and networking.*

10. ***Enjoy the present moment.*** *Present time consciousness means living one day and one moment at a time. The word happiness comes from the root word meaning to happen. Happiness comes from fully living in the present moment and recognizing that each action takes you down one fork at a crossroad.*

11. ***Don't look back too much.*** *An occasional analysis of the past reveals trends and lessons. For the most part, however, don't relive past decisions and second-guess yourself. Live in the present moment and stay alert for new possibilities.*

12. ***Simplify.*** *Energy blocks and stagnation occur when your office and home are too cluttered. Clear out the accumulated junk and notice how your life feels lighter and more flowing. Excellent books are available on the Eastern art of feng shui and simplifying your life.*

Love Yourself

Life is for learning. A baby learns to walk by first crawling, then falling repeatedly. Similarly, we all make mistakes and learn by trial and error. Ideally, we learn from our mistakes quickly and don't hurt others along the way. But no one is perfect. Sometimes we don't know which road to take and later wish we had chosen differently.

Remembering you were once a little baby helps you love and forgive yourself. Post a baby picture of yourself where you'll see it to remind yourself that you're still learning to walk in some areas of your life. Realize that you're not the only one who has made mistakes.

This is not a rationalization for inappropriate living, but the basis for *self-forgiveness* that transforms you into a highly functioning human being. Your brain processes over 50,000 thoughts and feelings daily. Is it any wonder that you may have an occasional and transient negative thought? Some people don't realize this and punish themselves because they feel lowly and evil.

I once counseled a young mother who thought she was going crazy after being up night after night with her sick, crying baby. Tired and frazzled, she momentarily thought how much easier her life would be if her baby died. Those thoughts horrified her and filled her with anxiety despite no plan or intention to act on her thought. Her feelings were *warning signals* that she was overstressed and fatigued. How many others have similarly carried a burden around with them and needlessly felt guilt and self-loathing?

During a serious life crisis, it's fairly common to have temporary thoughts of wanting to give up and die. These are *red flags* that you need a break and outside help. Thoughts like this are indications that you are hurting and want to ease the pain. Don't think you're crazy or immoral for having such thoughts, but do take them seriously. When your burdens seem too heavy to bear, contact a holistic health care physician, professional counselor, and minister or spiritual advisor.

I mention *holistic health* care here because many so-called 'mental' symptoms are due to ***nutritional deficiencies, spinal cord pressure, and blocked emotions.*** While working as a clinical psychologist, I thought that 'talk therapy' and, when necessary, psychiatric medications were the only solutions for psychological problems.

Now, thanks to many clinical successes using holistic health care, I know that the three causes above can create a variety of symptoms including depression, panic attacks, nervousness, suicidal feelings, obsessive-compulsive disorder, and more.

To consistently have positive thoughts, words, and deeds is an ideal to aspire toward, but don't flagellate yourself when you fall short. When you make a mistake, *apologize, make amends, and do better the next time.* That's what the word *repent* originally meant. As

Oliver Wendell Holmes said, "The greatest thing in the world is not so much where we stand, as in what direction we are moving."

Death wishes, angry thoughts, sexual experimentation, periodic discontent and reevaluation of one's life are all common in the course of a lifetime. Have you ever experienced poor self-image, sexual concerns, family problems, or a perceived lack of parental attention? So have most people at one time or another. You don't have to punish yourself because of imperfect life choices in the past. Strive for saintly living, but don't beat yourself up when you fall short of the mark.

In my years of counseling others, I learned that most of us go through similar problems during various stages in life. It's called *your story.* The question is, are you going to play out that old sad story endlessly, or create a more happy and positive one?

This is so crucial that I'll say it again. Don't let past thoughts, words, or deeds keep you from loving, accepting, and forgiving yourself and others. Everyone makes mistakes. Maturation often involves trial and error learning. Make a distinction between the *doer and the deed:* you may have acted badly in the past, but that doesn't make you a bad person.

Everyone is unique and it's healthy to march to your own drummer. People vary greatly in age, color, size, shape, sexual orientation, religious beliefs, cultural norms, hair and clothing styles, and other criteria. The strength and beauty of humanity lies, in part, in the rich variation among individuals. Don't waste time trying to emulate a nonexistent 'normal' pattern. Love Creator, yourself, and others, then live how you think is best.

Trust Your Inner Wisdom

Another key to heightened awareness is getting in touch with your innate intelligence. *Listening to your gut* and *following your hunches* are other ways of describing this phenomenon. No one knows you like you know yourself. Yes, there's a time to consult loved ones, but also trust your own instincts. Shakespeare said, "Our doubts are traitors, and make us lose the good we oft might win, by fearing to attempt."

Trusting yourself is a giant step toward achieving total success.

In addition to your educated mind, you have a remarkable transcendent source of consciousness. As the musician Sting says, "Let your soul be your pilot, let your soul guide you, it'll guide you well."

Your feelings indicate whether you're getting closer or further from the life of your dreams. In *Ask and It Is Given,* Esther and Jerry Hicks teach this "Law of Attraction" concept very well. Simply put, *your emotional guidance system* tells you:

1. *your thoughts, words and deeds are aligned with Source and your highest visions (you feel happy, positive and energized)*
2. *your life is out of sync with your highest visions and you've forgotten who you are (you feel sad, negative and tired)*

In this bustling material world, some people aren't in touch with their inner knowing. They tune out their soul's pleading for creativity, play, quiet, space, peace, purpose, and growth. There's a better way. Trust your inner guidance to cultivate greater awareness about what is best for you.

Ventilation

To ventilate means to bring in the fresh and put out the stale. Most of us have experienced sadness, anger, guilt, resentment, hurt, and embarrassment. If kept inside, these emotions can contribute to physical and emotional ailments.

Denise was a sixty-year-old counselor who worked on herself over the years using different psychological methods. However, she still suffered with physical and emotional symptoms and sought my help to balance herself. Using an emotional release technique, I found feelings associated with 'kill' and 'depression' occurring at age six.

I hesitated to tell her this information since I couldn't imagine a six-year-old with those emotions, but I had learned to trust the technique.

When I shared this with Denise, she turned pale and said, "Oh, my God, that's still affecting me?"

She explained that she really wanted a pony when she was six years old and her grandpa bought her one. While unloading bales of hay to feed it, he suffered a heart attack and died. Denise's grandmother, who wasn't very mentally balanced, told her that she (Denise) killed her grandpa. "If you didn't want that pony, he would still be alive." Denise spent most of her youth feeling depressed because she really believed she killed him.

Seventy-year-old Otto suffered with severe abdominal symptoms for nearly sixty years. Despite many medical tests and treatments, his constant pain and bowel problems continued. My analysis showed that *emotional blocks* were part of the cause. I found fear of death at the age of ten causing panic feelings, but Otto denied having any past emotional trauma. I made an adjustment and suggested that he might remember something from the past.

The next visit, Otto told me he had nightmares the night of his last office visit. The next day he remembered that at the age of ten, he came home from school and found his house burning to the ground. He didn't know if any family members were inside. They weren't but it was extremely traumatic to him. A month later, his mother gave birth to a boy but the baby died soon after.

No past emotional trauma?

Regularly releasing pent up stress is essential for true wellness.

Get things *off your chest* so you can see life more clearly. Let go of negative feelings about past events so they don't overly influence your present moments. Dr. Wayne Dyer described the past as like the wake from a boat. The wake doesn't drive the boat, you do. Stay focused on what's ahead and *don't look back* too much.

Difficult times are part of living on planet earth. However, it's not the external event but *your internal response* that determines how you come through stressful challenges. Thus, the wise develop strategies such as ventilation for releasing emotional baggage.

The following approaches can often assist releasing stuck emotions: Neuro-emotional Technique, Emotional Freedom Technique, Koren Specific Technique, the Sedona Method Release Technique, and Neuro-Linguistic Programming.

Other recommendations for ventilation include:

- ***Prayer** reminds you that you're not alone in this journey. Guidance and assistance always and abundantly flow from Life Source and Higher Energy Assistance especially when you are open to it. The best prayers are those of gratitude since blessings endlessly shine down on all.*
- ***Counseling** is another way to rid yourself of negative emotions. Seek professional help if your situation is severe or if self-improvement techniques don't help. Don't be embarrassed to seek guidance from mental health professionals or pastoral counselors. Most people have occasional life crises that require outside help. Knowing when to get outside help is a sign of strength, not weakness.*
- ***Catharsis** techniques are great ways to release stress. Native Americans had a unique method of releasing negative inner emotions: they dug a hole in the ground, yelled their problems into the hole, then filled the hole back up. Emotions released, no negative side effects, no expense.*

  Other techniques involve holding a pillow over your mouth and screaming out pent up emotions. Use your hands or a whiffle ball bat to beat up a pillow or cushion. Write your concerns in the sand by the water's edge and watch the waves erase them.
- ***Writing out concerns** also helps. Seeing your problems on paper makes them seem more manageable. Write out your negative emotions, then tear up or burn the paper to complete the release. Or list all your problems and all your blessings and see which list is longer.*

- ***Self-talk** is another simple but effective technique. Take a walk and talk to yourself: "OK, I have this problem. How can I release the negativity? What are my choices for improvement?" Use an old Dale Carnegie tip and consider, "What is the very worst that could happen in this situation? If the very worst did happen, what would I do?" Talking through the worst case scenario, which rarely happens, helps you release fears and generate positive options.*

- ***Keep an open mind.** Don't limit yourself by believing only what you were taught in your youth. Keep a healthy open-minded skepticism when examining new ideas, products, and services. When I first heard about yoga at age sixteen, my first response was a moronic: "You mean like Yogi Bear?" Over time, I felt moved to explore yoga and meditation and the quality of my life increased greatly.*

- ***Avoid worrying.** Excessive worry causes physical and emotional problems. Denis Waitley PhD points out that of all your worries, usually about 60% are unwarranted, 20% are in the past, and 10% are petty. Of the remaining 10%, only half of them are really significant and you can't do anything about half of that 5%. Thus, only 2% of your worries are real, substantial, and under your control. The take away? Focus on the things you can change and don't let the other 98% cloud your mind.*

- ***Share your skeletons.** Discuss your deep dark secrets with those you trust. Self-disclosure has tremendous curative value and helps you forgive yourself and others. I don't recommend excessive complaining, but sharing valid concerns with those who care helps immensely. Sidney Jourard PhD, author of The Transparent Self, recommended intimate sharing as a primary technique for releasing inner negative content.*

  As part of my master's training in clinical psychology, I went through two years of group and individual psychotherapy. Like all of us, I had feelings, thoughts and actions that I wasn't proud of or comfortable with. As I shared these in counseling sessions, I experienced a profound relief and release. From the group and therapists, I received consensual validation, that is, most people have similar experiences. Consider opening up to others as a tremendous way of ventilating.

- ***Holistic Breathing Technique** involves deep, open-mouth, noisy, and prolonged diaphragmatic breathing. It's no coincidence that in*

> *some cultures, Aramaic and Oriental, for example, the words breath and spirit were interchangeable. This technique releases stress and anxiety and makes stuck energy more available for present moment living. Other excellent breathing techniques have been taught by Stan Grof MD, Jacquelyn Small LMSW, Tom Goode ND, and Rusty Barrier PhD.*

Quieting the Rational Mind

The philosopher Cicero said, "Only the person who is relaxed can create, and to that mind ideas flow like lightning."

On an evolutionary timeline, the cerebral cortexes are fairly new innovations. These twin computers have amazing abilities, but most people haven't learned how to control them. Thus the saying, "The mind is a wonderful servant but a horrible master." Many people suffer from incessant thinking, worrying, and reminiscing. Excessive mental activity blocks clear awareness and all the accompanying benefits.

The brain has been compared to a drunken monkey that thinks it's the master of the house. It runs around, chattering constantly and acting like a fool. This creates a lot of noise and may even be entertaining for a time. In the long run, though, the house becomes a mess and uninhabitable.

Another analogy compares the brain with a wild elephant that charges around at will and destroys everything in its path. The elephant/brain needs to be tamed and more available for doing useful work.

The brain is so active that most of us perceive life one or more thoughts away from the real experience. We're thinking: "I'm eating now; I'm playing with the kids now; I'm working now" and so on instead of fully enjoying the moment. An *overly active* mind constantly labels and monitors experiences so that we may never fully enjoy the real event.

How can you quiet your brain and increasingly become the master of your life? Here's a hint: watch children at play and observe their *total involvement in the moment.*

Many powerful centering techniques can calm the brain and help you stay in the present moment. Simply take a little time each day to get quiet within. Do activities that you enjoy and help you feel clear and peaceful. The key is to *enjoy just being* for a while without worrying, analyzing or otherwise dissecting the experience.

Ways to dampen the brain's frenzied activity include: spend time in nature, listen to music, play with pets and children, garden, read, make love, watch a great movie or play, soak in a hot tub, exercise, meditate, do yoga, enjoy time with loved ones, serve others, study topics of interest, pray, cook, sew, sunbathe, relax in a hammock, or other ways to become absorbed in life's golden present moments.

You deserve to feel happy, peaceful and enthusiastic. Let those precious feelings carry over into your other life activities. This helps counteract the feeling that life is a hectic, hopeless, and endless rat race.

Here are a few simple relaxation techniques. Because meditation is so important, I'll discuss that in a separate section.

Relaxation methods such as *Jacobsen's progressive contraction relaxation technique* can be mastered with a little practice. Lie down or sit comfortably in a quiet place while breathing slowly and deeply. Progressively tighten and then relax the major muscle groups by first contracting the muscles of the feet and legs. Hold that tightness for a few seconds before letting all the tension go. Let your muscles feel completely relaxed, warm, and heavy.

Then alternately tighten the muscles of the buttocks, abdomen and lower back, chest and upper back, hands and arms, shoulders, and neck. To relax facial muscles: raise the eyebrows high for the forehead muscles; close your eyes tightly for cheek and eye muscles; clench the jaw tightly for jaw muscles.

From that point on, let your mouth part open slightly as you breathe slowly and deeply. Then take inventory of your body. If any area still feels tense, repeat the contraction and relaxation there until your entire body feels deeply and pleasantly relaxed. Enjoy that relaxed state for several minutes or longer if you like.

With practice, you will quickly notice the difference between tension and relaxation and be more aware when you tense up during the day. You can then simply take a few deep breaths and release the anxiety while thinking: "All my muscles feel completely relaxed, warm, and heavy."

Over time, your body and brain will stay relaxed throughout the day *despite outward stresses.* Remember, it's not what is going on around you that creates your reality. You can't control that. It's your *internal state of being* and you can always control that.

Another technique involves *touching forehead reflex points* to calm stress and reach deep relaxation. These reflex points can be felt as bumps or knobs a few inches directly above the eyebrows. Touch these points lightly with the pads of your three middle fingers of each hand. Use the technique twice a day for five minutes. The middle of the day and just before bedtime are good times for most people.

While touching these points, you have a number of options. First, you can just watch your thoughts go by, but not be attached to them. You can pray or think of happy times in your life. Or you can actively think about any worries and fears. In general, I don't recommend that but you can *productively process problems* while touching the forehead points.

Those reflex points apparently activate deep centers in the brain that assist *reaching acceptance or generating alternative solutions.* Touching the forehead points helps clarify whether it is a problem that must be accepted, or one that can be changed. If the situation can be changed, what are the best options or alternatives?

A final relaxation technique is to imagine *exhaling the negative and inhaling the positive.* Sit or lie down in a quiet setting with your eyes closed. Pray and intend to release all negativity while filling yourself with positive energies. As you *exhale,* release sadness, fear, guilt, anger, doubt, and other lower energy emotions. At the same time, visualize or feel a dark cloud leaving your body. Do this for 5 or 10 exhalations.

Then focus on higher energy emotions as you *inhale.* Imagine breathing in love, joy, peace, enthusiasm, and gratitude. At the same time, visualize your entire body filling with a warm, glowing golden-white light. Then give thanks for higher energy assistance and commit to sharing that love and light always and in all ways.

Meditation

Meditation confers many powerful holistic benefits. It's high on my list of practices that provide an inordinate amount of benefit for the time involved.

Alan Watts, in his book *Meditation,* stated: 'Most of us think compulsively all the time. If I think all the time, I'm living entirely in the world of symbols and I'm never in relationship with reality. The difference between myself and all the rest of the universe is nothing more than an idea, it is not a real difference. Meditation is a way in which we come to feel our basic inseparability from the whole universe. By going out of your mind you come to your senses.'

A Harvard *Spirituality and Healing* conference noted: "For more than 25 years, laboratories at the Harvard Medical School have systematically studied the benefits of mind/body interactions. This research has shown that when a person engages in a repetitive prayer, word, sound or phrase—and when intrusive thoughts are passively disregarded—specific physiologic changes ensue. Metabolism, heart rate, and breathing frequency all decrease and distinctive slower brain waves appear."

Further, "These changes are exactly the opposite of those induced by stress and can help reduce hypertension, palpitations, insomnia, infertility, premenstrual syndrome, chronic pain and the symptoms of cancer and AIDS. In fact, to the extent that any disease is caused or made worse by stress, to that extent is this physiological state an effective therapy."

Regarding the benefits of meditation, Paramahansa Yogananda wrote, "Why should you think He is not everywhere? The air is filled with music that is caught by the radio – music that otherwise you would not know about. And so it is with God. He is with you every minute of your existence, yet the only way to realize this is to meditate."

Father Thomas Keating stated, "Silence is the language God speaks, and everything else is a bad translation." French physicist, mathematician, and philosopher Blaise Pascal said, "All man's miseries derive from not being able to sit quietly in a room alone."

Meditation, anyone?

Classes are taught at many colleges, health facilities, enlightened churches, and holistic retreats or seminars. With regular practice, learning to meditate is easy. There are several methods I can recommend from personal experience:

- *Transcendental Meditation™ taught by Maharishi Mahesh Yogi*
- *Kriya Yoga taught by The Self Realization Fellowship and founded by Paramahansa Yogananda*
- *Integral Hatha Yoga taught by Sri Swami Satchidananda*

These also teach yoga postures and breathing techniques that I have used for many years. I also recommend the practices described in Peter Kelder's book *Ancient Secret of the Fountain of Youth.*

Recommended books on the subject include *Journey of Awakening: A Meditator's Guidebook* by Ram Dass; *The Varieties of the Meditative Experience* by Daniel Goleman PhD; and *Beyond Biofeedback* by Elmer Green PhD and Alyce Green.

One general meditation technique involves working with the breath and/or sound while you sit quietly with eyes closed. Focus your awareness at the tip of your nose as you breathe in and out deeply but gently at a rate that is comfortable for you. With each exhalation, you can silently repeat a mantra or word that has spiritual significance.

Recommended mantras include the creational and manifesting sounds OM and AH. Depending on your spiritual path, you may want to use names for the Light that contain the 'AH' sound: God, Allah, Buddha, Ram, Wanka Tanka or Krishna. Others are Peace, One, Great Spirit, OM Shanti (Sanskrit for Divine peace), Shalom (Jewish for peace), Jesus or any other word that reminds you of Divine Oneness.

Use the mantra in three phases: aloud for a few repetitions, then more quietly until just moving the lips without sound, and then silently. For beginning meditators, mentally repeat the mantra with each exhalation. Later, you can use the mantra only when you find yourself thinking too much or getting drowsy.

If you become aware of your brain thinking too much, quietly return your focus to the breathing and mantra. Don't chastise yourself; meditation should be an effortless and gentle process. While meditating, your computer brain may generate many reasons why you should be doing something else. Like the wild elephant, it may temporarily become even more agitated after initially being chained.

At first, meditation may seem like a practice in self-discipline. In time, however, your mind will naturally gravitate toward becoming more clear, peaceful, and blissful. This level of consciousness can eventually generalize into *your normative state.*

Components of successful meditation include:

- *Find a quiet spot where you won't be bothered by phones, excessive noise, or other interruptions.*
- *Program yourself to ignore any outside noises.*
- *Some teachers recommend doing meditation at dawn and dusk. Others recommend just before lunch and dinner when your stomach is empty and you are somewhat fatigued or stressed.*

- *Sit with the spine straight. For some, a half or full lotus position works well. A pillow or two under the buttocks assists a proper upright posture in this position. For others, sitting on a chair with feet on the floor is more comfortable.*
- *Place your hands on your thighs or in your lap with palms up.*
- *Use diaphragmatic breathing. Let the abdomen move downward and outward as you inhale; gently pull the abdominal muscles upward and inward as you exhale.*
- *Breathe at a slow, rhythmic pace through the nostrils. Breathing through the mouth causes dryness that may interfere with a peaceful experience.*
- *Let the jaw and facial muscles relax completely with your lips parted slightly.*
- *With eyes closed, shift your focus on the sixth chakra, the spiritual third eye just above the bridge of the nose.*
- *Let the breath and/or mantra proceed naturally and effortlessly.*
- *Meditate for 15 to 20 minutes but don't set an alarm. Open one eye to check a clock when you feel the time has elapsed.*
- *Sit quietly for a few moments before arising.*

Remember to be patient and continue meditating every day. Soon it will become a highlight of your day, an oasis of tranquility amidst life's hectic demands. A subtle but important distinction will also become apparent: thoughts may still come and go, but you'll be in touch with the part of yourself that isn't doing the thinking. Thoughts will drift through like fleecy clouds instead of incessant static. Just watch them pass by.

Any subject that surfaces often during meditation may indicate an imbalance that needs attention. Layers of negative thinking and repressed emotions may be released over time. Inspirational ideas may come to your attention. I keep a notepad by my meditation area so I can jot down new insights *after* the session.

Reprogramming Your Brain

Another approach to expanding your awareness involves *positively reprogramming* your biocomputer. First century philosopher Epictetus said, "Men are disturbed not by things, but by the views which they take of them." As discussed, it's not the outside event that affects your feelings, but *what you tell yourself* about it. Improving how you talk, think, and act changes how you feel.

If you begin to feel depressed or upset, think back to what you just thought or said. What did you tell yourself? If your date stands you up, you could think, "We must not have been suited for each other" versus "No one will ever love me." If you spill a glass of water, you could think, "Accidents happen" instead of "I'm such a klutz. I always mess up!"

Your language and beliefs shape your actions and destiny. You likely have old *unconscious negative scripts* – bits and pieces of limiting programming that aren't really true. These negative internal dialogues can effectively hypnotize you into a confused and disempowered being.

Those committed to reaching their highest potential will want to reprogram their inner tapes. Here's a personal example of how beliefs and the accompanying language shape reality. As a youth, I wasn't very mechanically oriented and would sometimes make statements like, "I was born with two left thumbs" or "I'm just not good at this type of work." Those words and beliefs became my self-fulfilling prophecy and my reality.

One day, my dad said something that affected my way of thinking.

I asked how he was so good at carpentry, electrical work, mechanics, and other skills. He thought a moment and replied, "I always felt that if someone put it together, I could take it apart, figure out how it works and fix it." The power and simplicity of his statement went to my core. I consciously began to think, speak, and act differently about my ability to perform mechanical tasks.

To put myself through graduate school, I worked at a number of jobs that required manual dexterity and did well. Today, I enjoy repairing things around the house. It's fun, challenging, and feels good to be self-sufficient.

Watch for put down thoughts or statements and ask others to help you become more aware of negative self-talk. Whenever you become aware of a negative expression, refute it and replace it with a more appropriate one. For example, if asked to perform a difficult task, you might automatically think, "I know I'll blow it. I always do." Instead, immediately create a more positive tape such as, "I am improving in this area. I can do it."

In *Healthy Pleasures,* David Sobel MD and Robert E. Ornstein PhD list common erroneous ways of thinking to avoid:

- *Am I thinking in all-or-none terms?*
- *Am I assuming every situation is the same?*
- *Am I confusing a rare occurrence with a high probability?*
- *Am I assuming the worst possible outcome?*
- *Am I overlooking my strengths?*
- *Am I blaming myself for something beyond my control?*
- *Am I expecting perfection in myself and others?*
- *How could I have handled this situation differently?*
- *What difference will this make in a week, a year, or 10 years?*

Consider these questions and *start now* to reprogram your mind more positively. Remember, your brain follows the instructions you put into your biocomputer. With practice, you'll feel better about yourself and improve your performance in every area of life. Since you're the author of your own life story, why not write an exciting adventure with a happy ending?

Another suggestion for more conscious language is to remove the words: "I'll try, I can't, I should, and maybe I could." Instead, use: "I'll do it, there's always a way, I choose to, and I know I can." Also *avoid global statements* and false generalizations such as "*no one* likes me, *everyone* has it better than me, you *always* put me down, or the world is a *total* mess."

Asking great questions is another key to greater awareness. Many people repetitively ask bad questions that reinforce their problem. For example, a depressed person might frequently ask, "Why am I tired and down all the time?" Since we tend to move toward our most dominant thoughts, it's best to ask questions that trigger positive solutions. A better question would be, "How can I feel more energetic and happy now and every day?" Then your awesome computer-brain will set out to solve that question.

Recommended reading for more information about this topic includes: *A Guide to Rational Living* by Ellis and Harper; *Reframing: NeuroLinguistic Programming and the Transformation of Meaning* by Grinder and Bandler; *Unlimited Power* by Tony Robbins; *A Handbook for Higher Consciousness* by Ken Keyes; and *Woulda, Coulda, Shoulda: Overcoming Regrets, Mistakes, and Missed Opportunities* by Freeman and Dewolf.

Awareness and Children

Raising children with love, respect, and awareness is an important key so they and future generations are healthy, happy, and fulfilled.

When children become unruly or unhappy, *consider common causes first:* Are they hungry and experiencing low blood sugar? Are they tired? Are they upset or fearful about something? Are they ill or in pain? Little ones communicate with crying, behavior changes, and mood swings. Ask them what is wrong and check the above categories before judging their behavior as "just being bad." Growth spurts can be physically and emotionally exhausting and may engender temporary "bratty" behavior.

Children are very impressionable so *closely monitor their mental input*. Limit TV viewing to entertaining and educational programs primarily on public TV stations. Avoid shows with negativity, violence, and frequent commercials for sugary and junk foods. Don't let young children watch graphic video games, news, and other shows. Denis Waitley PhD says: "Most of what is available on TV is junk food that leads to mental malnutrition and poor emotional and spiritual health."

By the time children finish high school, they have seen 15,000 hours of television and 30,000 incidents of violence and aggression. A Michigan State University study showed that the average fourteen-year-old watches 1400 sexual acts or references to sexual acts on TV each year. Researchers concluded, "There's little indication that parents exercise any control, positive or negative, over TV viewing by teens."

Here's an example of the importance of awareness with children. A twelve-year-old boy was brought to my office for holistic health care. Steven had been diagnosed with ADHD (Attention Deficit Hyperactivity Disorder) and was taking four medications. His symptoms included behavioral outbursts, insomnia, obesity, poor grades and difficulty focusing.

His history revealed the following:

1. *The behavioral outbursts were frequent at home with his mom, mild and occasional at school, and never around his dad.*
2. *Lots of sugary junk foods—candy, pastries, and pop—were all he eats."*
3. *He never exercised.*
4. *He spent most of his time playing video games and watching movies or TV—all with violent themes.*

No health care providers had even inquired about these details.

Steven was just put on four drugs.

I recommended a holistic treatment program that included:

- *Reduction in sweets and increase in healthy food and water*
- *Nutritional supplements for overall health and support of brain and adrenal glands*
- *Behavior modification techniques to extinguish inappropriate behaviors at home and reinforce healthier ones*
- *Mild exercise such as walking*
- *Only nonviolent computer games and TV on a limited basis*

I wish I could tell you how well that program worked, but they didn't return after the second visit. I heard through other family members that Steven raised such a ruckus over the program that his mom gave in. Too bad. He needs parental guidance and holistic health care at this critical time in his life, not four medications.

Please don't let a lack of awareness cause preventable problems for the young ones in your life.

Many wise elders I've talked with share their concerns that today's youth are often exempt from helping with work at home. Having work responsibilities early in life is important for developing cooperation and maturity. Today's parents sometimes make it too easy for their children, thereby denying important lessons about integrity and teamwork.

The plant world provides an excellent analogy. If a plant has it too easy and is watered too often, a shallow root system results. The healthiest plants have to *struggle a little* and thus put down a deep root system. This firm foundation keeps it rooted during windy days and makes tall growth possible. In the same way, graduated levels of work and responsibility help youngsters learn important lessons that serve them throughout their lifetimes.

Elders also stress the importance of enjoying children while they are young because in a blink of an eye they'll be grown. Take time to enjoy precious moments with little ones while you can. Expose them to positive art, music, literature and wisdom sources. Children are like sponges, always ready to soak up incoming information. Make those messages inspirational and positive.

Children are sensitive so treat them gently, but with firm guidelines and tough love. Be a good model for healthy and balanced behavior. Watch what you say and do around them since children learn by example. Maintain the perspective that every one is heaven's special child in our care for a short time to cherish, nurture, and learn from.

Recommended reading for optimally raising children includes: *Toddlers and Parents* by T. Barry Brazelton MD; *How To Raise A Healthy Child* by Robert Mendelsohn MD; *The Mother is the Baby's First Guru* by S.S. Satchidananda; *The Early Childhood Years* by Theresa and Frank Caplan; *What Do You Really Want For Your Children?* by Wayne Dyer EdD; and *Raising Positive Kids In A Negative World* by Zig Ziglar.

Aging

How would you feel and act if you didn't know how old you are?

Keys to enjoying a long and vital life include thinking young, taking great care of yourself, and staying active. Exuberant health into the senior years is possible but requires increased attention to special needs. As Ben Douglas MD stated in *Ageless: Living Younger Longer,* "You can live younger longer; we can all choose to age less and enjoy a longer, healthier life."

Your biological age is different than your chronological age. You have much control over how long and how well your body functions. Forget the clichés that it's all downhill after 40. In truth, it's all downhill when you think it is. Bea, a local yoga teacher, said she felt 80 years old when she starting doing yoga at age 60, but when she reached 80, she felt like she was 40.

As your body ages, treat it like a vintage car that needs extra care and maintenance. As Peter Kelder wrote in *Fountain of Youth,*

"If an old person truly wants to grow younger, they must think, act and behave like a younger person, and eliminate the attitudes and mannerisms of old age."

An enlightened awareness is crucial here. Aging isn't bad, it's just different. Develop a perspective that recognizes the beauty in each stage of life. Work to keep your physical body as healthy as possible for as long as you can. As time wears down the bodily vehicle, though, don't fret. Each phase of life has its importance and purpose.

Advanced age is exquisitely designed to impart benefits that often elude younger, more active people. Elders can learn important lessons that make bodily degeneration eminently worthwhile. As the body slows down, seniors naturally experience more meditation-like reveries.

As the five senses lose their clarity, *extrasensory perceptions* such as sensing 'departed' loved ones can increase.

Do you excessively mourn over your old cars that have worn out? How about the clothes you wore fifty years ago? Of course not. How silly, then, to bemoan the aging of a physical shell that houses your enduring self for a mere fraction of eternity. I know this is easier said than done when it's happening to you, but it is possible.

Elders have helped us in many ways. As they prepare to transition from this life, they deserve our love, respect, and time. Rather than sedating them in substandard nursing homes, let's provide optimal environments for graduating into the next life experience.

For more information about aging, death, and dying, read books by Elisabeth Kubler-Ross MD, Herman Feifel PhD, and other gerontology and thanatology authors. *Life's Finishing School: Conscious Living, Conscious Dying* by Helen Ansley is especially recommended.

Avoid Energy Disturbers

Maintaining optimal awareness is easier when your energy is high and harmonious. It's more difficult when others are disrupting your energy. The most likely person who is disturbing your energy is you. We've already discussed the law of attraction and importance of focusing on gratitude, peace, joy, love, and enthusiasm.

I also watch out for others who aren't aware of their negative impact. Have you ever talked with someone and felt depressed or fatigued afterwards? They may be energy drainers. Tips for handling this include:

1. *if they overly focus on negative topics, divert the conversation to positive ones*
2. *if they rehash "ain't it awful" stories, initiate a walk or other pleasant activity*
3. *if they go overboard about their health problems, shift the conversation to how both of you can improve your lives*
4. *if numbers 1 through 3 fail, be assertive and tell them you don't want to hear excessive negativity. If they persist, leave.*

Norman Shealy MD, PhD, author and founder of the American Holistic Medical Association, says we need to shield ourselves from people who are *sappers and zappers.* Sappers are usually depressed and try to soak up the energy from others. No matter what you do for a sapper, it's not enough. Zappers are indiscriminately angry and send off negative energy toward others. To shield yourself from such people, cross your arms over your chest and abdominal area, or walk away.

Before meditating or praying, affirm that you are shielded with love and light. Imagine golden white or violet light pouring outward from the solar plexus area to form a shield that protects you from negativity, evil, and darkness. Visualize this light extending all around your body and forming a protective bubble or cocoon.

Limit all sources of negative input. If any group or club focuses too much on lower energy topics, avoid them. Especially be aware if they want to control your mind and lighten your pocketbook. As Walt Whitman said two centuries ago, "Reexamine all you have been told at school or church, or in any books, and dismiss whatever insults your own soul."

Avoid listening to music with lyrics that brainwash you to think disempowering themes such as you can't live without a certain person in your life. When I was in high school, popular songs conveyed limiting messages such as, "I can't live without you, my life is empty without you." When my first love dumped me, guess what? I believed those lyrics and it took me a long time to realize there were good reasons for the demise of our relationship.

Recent research has demonstrated that *negative TV viewing* increases sadness and anxiety among viewers who internalize observed stresses. Whatever the source, negativity can de-energize, distort, depress, or overstimulate so *monitor your input.*

Spending quality time in nature releases accumulated negative energies. To better handle life's unavoidable stresses, regularly walk in nature and enjoy the beauty. Practice energy enhancing techniques such as yoga, tai chi and qi gong.

Universal energy or chi is said to be more abundant where the sky, sun, wind, water, or earth meet. Shuffling barefoot in water, grass, sand, or dirt removes negative energies and absorbs more positive, grounded ones. To learn more, visit ***Earthing.com***.

Shaking off negative energies is especially important for health care practitioners who work on diseased and tense individuals. Tingling and pressure in the hands and arms signal a need for shielding and shaking techniques. Shake your hands briskly as if you were trying to flip water off your hands. Wash your hands in cold water to help remove imbalanced energies.

The *Lion's Breath* is a breathing technique to release imbalanced energies. Take a deep breath in, then forcefully and quickly exhale through the opened mouth while sticking your tongue outward and downward. Repeat three times.

As always, *prevention* is the best approach. Use these various releasing and shielding techniques daily and more often when overstressed to protect yourself from lower, slower energies.

The Ripple Effect

The *Bhagavad-Gita,* a collection of Hindu wisdom teachings, says to do what you feel called to do and do it as well as you can, but don't be attached to the fruits of your actions.

A *ripple effect* emanates from your thoughts, words and deeds so don't get discouraged if you *don't seem* to be making the impact you want. Do your very best and know that is enough.

A personal lesson about this occurred many years ago when I gave my first holistic health seminar. The very reasonable admission fee went toward refurbishing our city's historic Majestic Theater. We publicized the event by radio, TV, newspaper and flyers and hoped for a full house of 300 people.

The big day arrived, ominously, as the first warm sunny day of spring in Ohio. Not a good sign. I figured maybe only 200 would attend because of the great weather. Show time approached and the crowd was very sparse but I still hoped for a late rush to reach the 100 mark.

Ten minutes *before* show time and only a handful of people were there. But hope springs eternal. Maybe the crowd had encountered heavy traffic or trouble parking in our small town? Maybe escaped wild animals were keeping the crowd at bay?

Ten minutes *past* starting time: only 15 people were there and half of them were friends and family members. I wanted to crawl away and never give seminars again. I felt humiliated and very discouraged. But the show must go on. I somehow did my best and made it to the intermission.

In the backstage bathroom, I was still in shock about the turnout. What could be worse? Wrong question to ask, I quickly found out. As I urinated forcefully, I discovered—to my horror—that my wireless microphone was still on. Maybe the audience didn't hear? I peeked through the curtain and saw my friends doubled over with laughter. They heard.

It *seemed like* one of the worst days in my life, a total failure.

I learned many lessons from that day – beside the obvious one about the microphone. We may not always reach the multitudes, but we can follow our inner calling and do our best. If we reach only one other person, who knows how far reaching those positive repercussions might be over time.

Here's an example.

One very special aftermath of my Majestic talk occurred with Ed, an audience member with terminal cancer. He became a patient after hearing my discussion of spiritual awareness and holistic health. His condition was too far advanced to respond to holistic health measures, but we had several fine talks about documented survival of consciousness after death.

After Ed passed on, I visited the funeral home. He was beloved by many and the line of visitors was long. Ed's wife, Jean, motioned for me to come up by the casket. It was the first time I line cut at a funeral, but she insisted. She proudly introduced me to her family and shared the following experience that occurred just before Ed's passing.

He had been in a coma for three days and was very near death when suddenly he became alert. Ed couldn't talk but he kept smiling and pointing out the window up to the sky. When Jean started to leave to get a drink of water, he hoarsely gasped: "Don't leave me." She reassured him that she would never leave. He smiled, pointed excitedly again toward the sky and said, "I love you," closed his eyes and passed on.

Jean felt that our talks had decreased Ed's fears, prepared him spiritually, and assisted his wonderful transition experience. So was my Majestic talk a flop or a grand slam homerun? Remember, you can't judge the ripple effect of your actions from a limited earthly perspective. Perform your heartfelt missions to the best of your ability and don't waste time judging the outcome.

Goal Setting

Enjoying radiant wellness requires a clear *awareness of what you want* and an unstoppable determination to reach your goals. Many high achievers attribute their success to following this principle. Regularly focus on your goals with gratitude and enthusiasm to set formidable forces into motion.

Alexander Graham Bell spoke of a *conquering force* within each of us: "What this power is, I cannot say. All I know is that it exists... and it becomes available only when you are in that state of mind in which you know exactly what you want... and are fully determined not to quit until you get it."

Here's an example of the power of goal setting. In the 1953 Yale graduating class, only 3 percent had clear and specific goals written down. Twenty years later, those 3 percent scored superior on ratings of happiness in life and were worth more financially than the other 97 percent combined.

Sports commentator and former football coach Lou Holtz teaches the importance of goal setting. At age 28, he was unemployed and with their third child on the way, he said: "I don't think I've ever been any lower in my entire life. But my wife was supportive and she bought me a book about goal setting... The only reason I'm the head coach at Notre Dame is that I've had goals and I've had dreams. Deep down inside, you'd better have a dream and you'd better have a goal or things don't happen."

Clearly, goal setting can aid achievement of your potential. Unfortunately, most people spend more time planning their vacations than their lives. What are your goals? What do you want to achieve?

Write out your goals in the following areas: spiritual, physical, family, life work, psychosocial, and financial. List every goal that comes to mind, no matter how large or small, practical or seemingly impossible. The *sky's the limit* so let your self express all your inner dreams and goals.

Next, rewrite each goal using the following guidelines:

- ***Use present tense statements*** *as if it is already happening. For example, "I am making dollars per year, or I am a patient and loving parent" versus "I can or will…"*
- ***Be specific with dates, numbers, and wording:*** *"I weigh a trim 180 pounds by December 1, 2018" versus "I am losing weight." Or, "I lift weights and aerobically exercise three times per week" versus "I'm getting in good shape."*
- ***State what you want, not what you don't want.*** *Focus on the desired goal, not past undesirable habits. For example, "I enjoy breathing only fresh pure air and having healthy lungs" versus "I am smoking fewer cigarettes."*
- ***Use the 50/50 Rule of Belief.*** *Make your goals high enough to challenge you, but sufficiently within reach so you'll believe you can do it.*
- ***Remember the KISS Rule:*** *"Keep It Short and Simple." Don't combine two or more goals in the same sentence.*

Be sure to leave room for miracles and don't limit yourself. Some goal setting experts advise to just focus on the "what" and let Universe take care of the "how." That approach recognizes a Higher Power that assists in unexpected ways when we intently focus on our goals.

Read or say your goals the first thing in the morning and the last thing at night before sleeping. While doing so, be filled with *gratitude and enthusiasm,* two of the highest energy emotions that exist.

Realize that your goals are coming to you in the right way and at the right time. Hold the image that they are coming to you now to create a deep sense of thankfulness and excitement. Then take *inspired action steps* and stay alert for people and opportunities to assist the fulfillment of your goals.

By consistently setting and pursuing your goals, you redesign and shape your life for the better. As Thoreau put it, "If one advances confidently in the direction of his own dreams and endeavors, to lead the life which he has imagined, he will meet with a success unexpected in common hours."

Over time, it's good to change and even delete some goals. It's normal to change your priorities as you discover what is really important to you. After you reach your goals, reassess and plan your next steps. As Zig Ziglar teaches, the rule is: go as far as you can see. When you get there, look around and decide where you want to go next.

Affirmations are first cousins to goal setting and follow similar principles. Write out and post positive affirmations where you'll read them often. Repeated exposure to these lofty statements changes the way you view life and your potential. Suggested affirmations include:

- *Today is already a great day!*
- *I think only good thoughts and I feel wonderful!*
- *I am happy and enjoy life!*
- *I choose health, happiness, and total success!*

Don't forget Emil Coue's classic: "Everyday, in every way, I am getting better and better." Generate your own affirmations to fill yourself with positive expectancy.

Recommended books and tapes about the power of goal setting include: *It Works* by R.H.J., *New Age Thinking* by Louis Tice; *The Psychology of Winning* by Denis Waitley PhD; *Think and Grow Rich* by

Napoleon Hill; *Dare To Win* by Mark Victor Hansen; and *See You At The Top* by Zig Ziglar. Excellent books by Jerry and Esther Hicks and *The Secret* book and movie by Rhonda Byrne also teach about the law of attraction.

Loving Relationships

The older I get, the more I appreciate outstanding relationships. I deeply love my family and friends. Loved ones are worth their weight in gold and a key ingredient for radiant wellness.

Psychiatrist Karl Menninger MD said, "Love cures people. Both the ones who give it and the ones who receive it." Healthy relationships help us grow toward balance and enlightenment. A connection with another person is a sacred privilege to be appreciated and enjoyed. Like a garden, relationships need to be cultivated. Those who nourish and respect others gain flowering results.

You deserve to experience wonderful levels of love in your primary relationship and with all your family and friends. *Don't settle for anything else.*

A real sense of freedom and openness to growth occurs when another person deeply loves and accepts you. Loving relationships are a transformational practice in which both people see the highest potential in each other.

On this theme, Rev. Eric Butterworth writes in *Life Is for Loving:* "Love is not to be found. It consists not in *finding* the right person but in *becoming* the right person... True marriage comes about as two people sense and see in each other something of the divine potential that is always present beyond appearances. This leads to a mutual commitment to help each other mate with one's Godself."

During a life between lives session—a visit to celestial realms during deep hypnosis—one woman explained how it can be when two souls make love. She described it as a swirling of intermingled colors and energy. Whether enjoying that or a more physical type of lovemaking, it is described as a million times better than on earth.

That's one reason why sex without love is only a fraction of what can be. It takes a higher level of maturity and awareness to realize that. *Sacred lovemaking* is a powerful way to transform emotionally and spiritually as well as a wonderful way to feel alive and blissful.

With the increased availability of pornography, more people are developing sexual addictions. *Sexual integrity* issues affect everyone in the family – another reason to monitor what goes into your mind. Graphic lustful images especially influence people who may be predisposed to addictions.

The end result is lowered self-esteem, ruined relationships, and a debasement of lovemaking. In addition, the adult film industry is replete with exploitation of women, drug abuse, and sexually transmitted diseases.

As you go through stages in a healthy relationship, focus on the good in each other instead of amplifying the less desirable points. Most relationships periodically encounter tough times. Strong winds that bend, but don't break a tree can make it stronger and more flexible. Similarly, weathering temporary storms in relationships can make them deeper and richer.

I'm not, however, recommending an unending commitment to marriage in all situations. Some people barely tolerate each other in a marriage that was a mistake in the beginning. I've counseled people whose lives were in shambles after decades of an abusive and unloving union.

One elderly woman who was contemplating suicide confessed: "I haven't loved my husband for forty years, but we stayed together because that's what we were taught." The "we'll make it work if it kills us" attitude aptly describes the stress-related illnesses that predominate in long-term negative relationships.

If your relationship lacks harmony, do everything you can to save it. The costs of broken marriages, especially when children are involved, are devastating. Both people in the relationship may benefit marital counseling and marriage enrichment training.

But if a bond is *truly unhappy* after many years of working on a relationship, let it go and move on. Life is too short to live in an unfulfilling relationship. Continuing a facade for the sake of following social or religious convention is not worth it. Needless to say, no one should remain in an abusive relationship. Physically abused women may not get a second chance to escape. Mental abuse is just as bad due to the invisible emotional wounds that result.

When a relationship does end – by death or separation – remember that your heart can only be broken if it's closed and hardened. After a breakup or death, some people remain in a long self-imposed isolation. Go through a period of mourning, but keep your heart open and, when you're ready, find another partner. There's more than one fish in the sea and more than one soulmate for each of us.

The good news is that a relationship doesn't have to end just because one person has passed on. You can enjoy a different but very real *inter-dimensional relationship* with them. Many patients over the years have somewhat sheepishly admitted to carrying on a conversation with departed loved ones. There's no need to be embarrassed about this.

It's not crazy or foolish because, as we'll discuss in the last chapter, there's *convincing proof* that death is not an end, just a new beginning. You can *telepathically talk* with your loved ones, feel their presence, and—in the inner quiet of your heart—hear their gentle replies.

Recommended books for nourishing healthy relationships include: *Communication Magic and Creating Relationship Trust* by Susie and Otto Collins; *Spirit Centered Relationships* by Gay Hendricks PhD and Katie Hendricks PhD; *Life Is For Loving* by Rev. Eric Butterworth; *The Art of Loving* by Erich Fromm PhD; and *Love and Living, Loving, and Learning* by Leo Buscaglia PhD.

Meaningful Lifework

Another vitally important aspect of radiant wellness is to perform *meaningful life work.* The verb "perform" is an apt choice because living well is like an artistic endeavor. Making your life a work of art includes fulfilling lifework.

Some evidence indicates that your soul, ideally in alignment with Universal Intelligence, *chose missions* before it came to earth. Those are your heart's dreams, visions and callings. You have unique purposes, special talents to share.

Unfortunately, many hate their jobs or are unfulfilled by them. Continuing work that lacks meaning and interest can sap the vitality out of a person. Deepak Chopra MD says that Monday morning is the most common time for heart attacks and associates this with going to an unhappy job week after week.

The saying "my heart just wasn't into it" has energetic and health implications. *Following the path with heart* for your lifework is wise for holistic wellbeing.

Complete retirement isn't a good idea for most people. Men, especially, tend to die at a younger age when they don't have fulfilling work to do. Life flows best when we are *fully engaged in life,* of service to others, and sharing our special gifts and talents.

Europeans are less likely than Americans to completely retire. Instead, as they get older, they take more vacations, decrease the numbers of days worked per week and transition to different kinds of work. That makes sense to me. I also like the idea of a sabbatical, taking several months to a year off during the middle age years to reassess and recharge.

Meaningful lifework isn't limited to your job. Attending to your soul's missions is usually a multidimensional process. We each have numerous roles in life: family member, significant other, friend, employer or employee, church member, community participant, and balanced individual. Following your bliss doesn't mean forsaking all other roles and just focusing on one aspect.

Fulfilling your various roles can be challenging, but it's possible and an important part of radiant wellness. Making a commitment to pursue your dreams is a first step. Take the time to identify your calling and how best to get started. Some people have the circumstances and intestinal fortitude to make wholesale changes abruptly. Others may choose a more gradual transition over time. Whichever path you choose, start now!

At the same time, be wise about it. A Middle Eastern saying about this is: "Trust Allah, but tie up your camel." Daily living requires a certain income to survive so don't rush off and quit your day job prematurely. I know some people who did and wish they hadn't. Stay with your current work and expand your services until you *grow into* your higher calling.

To begin identifying your highest purpose, close your eyes, let yourself become relaxed, and ask for assistance from Life Source and your Higher Energy Assistants. Give thanks for guidance and clarity in realizing your highest calling in lifework and service to others. Then listen quietly for counsel from that *still small voice within.*

Let yourself dream for a moment, using your fullest imagination and passion, and answer this question: if you knew you could not fail, what would you do? Let the images flow and feel the excitement as, perhaps for the first time, you become aware of your special calling.

In the following exercise, *be aware of any clues* – words, pictures, feelings, symbols, colors, people, or places – that arise spontaneously. Answer the following questions by noting your very *first response:*

- *What are you naturally good at?*
- *What would you do if money were no object?*
- *What were your lifework dreams when you were a child?*
- *What service would you provide if you had only one year to live?*
- *What would you do without pay because you enjoy it so much?*
- *What do you read and talk about in your spare time?*
- *What gives you goose bumps, pressure over your chest, a lump in the throat, or tears in your eyes?*
- *How do you feel called to make this world a better place?*

Native Americans used a vision quest to help their young people identify and follow their special talents. Extended time in nature allowed getting in touch with Great Spirit and one's inner wisdom. If you're clueless about your lifework, take a few days and spend time near the woods, desert, mountains or water. Pray, meditate, write down insights that arise, and your dreams when you awaken. See what bubbles up. Then start moving in that direction.

Greater Awareness

You now have many new ideas and techniques for achieving increased awareness. Use this information to get ready for profound inner changes. Take time to cultivate your inner knowing that knows what to do in every situation. The benefits of your expanded intuition will be immeasurable.

As you face new decisions and challenges in life, remember that you always have the power to choose. Even in the face of tragedy and misfortune, you can always control your attitude. Focus on your strengths and the positive aspects of your life. With determination and creativity, there are always good options and solutions.

A verse from the *Dhammapada,* a collection of Buddhist teachings, states: "We are what we think. All that we are arises with our thought. With our thoughts we make the world. Speak and act with an impure mind and trouble will follow you as the wheel follows the ox that draws the cart... speak or act with a pure mind and happiness will follow you as your shadow, unshakable."

Within you – no matter what your current station in life – is infinite potential. Develop greater awareness so you'll know how to co-create the life of your dreams and make the world a better place.

The Bottom Line

The most important points in the *Awareness* chapter include:

1. *Make it a priority to increase your awareness for a richer life*
2. *Keep a positive perspective and stay open to the blessings amidst adversity*
3. *Love and forgive yourself and others since we all learn by trial and error*
4. *Develop your intuitive knowing and trust that inner wisdom*
5. *Embrace all of life, even the sad and bad times, and flow with the rhythms of change*
6. *Use ventilation techniques to release stress and frustration*
7. *Quiet your brain with relaxation, meditation and centering techniques*
8. *Use conscious language and expansive thoughts*
9. *Especially use awareness when dealing with children*
10. *Don't let yourself act like an old person but do recognize that aging is an integral part of life.*
11. *Shield yourself from energy sappers and zappers*
12. *Set goals, read them daily, and manifest them with enthusiasm and gratitude*
13. *Develop loving relationships with your significant other, family, and friends*
14. *Engage in meaningful life work and share your unique talents*

Action Steps for Increased Awareness

List two action steps you commit to starting within 30 days:

1. ______________________________
2. ______________________________

List two action steps you commit to starting within 60 days:

1. ______________________________
2. ______________________________

List two action steps you commit to starting within 90 days:

1. ______________________________
2. ______________________________

RADIANT

Natural Care

Key #6
Natural Care

Dean suffered with numbness and pain in his left hand and forearm. He consulted his medical doctor who referred him to a neurologist. That specialist ordered x-rays and an MRI of the neck that showed arthritis but no apparent cause of Dean's symptoms. Next, an electromyography test was performed that showed abnormal nerve transmission in the hand.

While he was waiting for the recommended medical treatment – probably carpal tunnel surgery – Dean came in for his scheduled chiropractic appointment. He told me about his symptoms and I checked for misalignment of the bones in his wrist. Several were out of normal alignment. I adjusted them and taped his wrist. I told him to take it easy with the wrist for a few days and let me know if he needed any follow-up care. No extra charge over the $35 fee for a spinal and skeletal tune-up.

A month later, I saw Dean and asked how his left hand was doing. "Oh, you fixed that right away. I didn't have any more symptoms after you adjusted it."

If he had sought natural health care first, he would have saved a lot of time and pain. And taxpayers – he was a state employee – would have saved a lot of money. If conservative measures didn't help, *then* the expensive tests and invasive surgery could be done. I see this situation nearly every day. Is there any wonder there's a national health care cost crisis? For a number of good reasons, more and more people are using *natural health care* to become radiantly well.

These approaches are more conservative and noninvasive than traditional medical ones. As such, natural methods have significantly fewer side effects and complications. They *work with the body* to restore normal function and are often very effective and less expensive.

Wise individuals *take responsibility* for their own health and make it a priority. They recognize that health is a precious commodity and do everything they can to maintain it. Those interested in wellness recognize that *symptoms are messages* from the body that something is awry. They seek to address *the core causes* of these symptoms with natural means whenever possible.

Julian Whitaker MD, who has promoted natural healing methods for decades, states: "Getting sick is neither natural nor unavoidable. We know that disease is often caused by the way we live, and by the food, water, and air we put into our bodies ...And we're finding that there are things we can do to not only avoid illness, but actually reverse it!

Your body is designed to heal itself naturally and then keep you healthy—IF you know how to help it!"

You only have one body during this earthly experience so it's smart to optimally care for it and *hold onto the original parts.* Once organs have been cut out, certain processes don't function normally. For example, the tonsils and adenoids are important parts of the immune system; the appendix houses beneficial intestinal bacteria; and the gall bladder stores and releases bile in a timely manner to break down ingested fats. Removing an organ often has adverse effects on other organs and systems.

Medications also change the function of bodily systems. Blocking acid production in the stomach interferes with mineral utilization and may lead to fragile bones. Weaker gastric juices can also allow 'bad' or pathogenic bacteria to over-colonize and cause inflammation of the intestines.

Drugs to decrease cholesterol to absurdly unhealthfully levels can adversely affect metabolic pathways that injure muscles and the liver. Increased deaths from *cardiomyopathy,* a disease of the heart muscle, have been reported since the introduction of cholesterol lowering drugs.

Davis was healthy and active, but was prescribed a cholesterol lowering drug by his medical doctor. This was done to supposedly protect his heart because of even though his levels were barely high by the new standards and perfect by norms used for decades.

His doctor didn't tell him that serious liver and muscle damage were two of the potential side effects. Soon, his heart muscle was severely damaged. Davis was told he would need five medications and probably a pacemaker. If that didn't help, he would need a heart transplant.

(Keep in mind that Davis was very healthy with no problems before following his medical doctors advice. Critics of the disease care system charge that it has become a *self-perpetuating industry* because the harm done in the name of health care.)

Davis had been a chiropractic patient of mine for many years, but I hadn't seen him for several months. I was shocked when his wife and daughter helped drag him in. His color was horrible and he could hardly talk. Not the strong and hardy Davis I had known. His ejection fraction, the percentage of blood pumped out of the heart with each beat, was only 25 percent, below the number required for hospice care.

I explained that his body might be able to repair itself if we removed the stressors and provided optimal nutrients. Davis and his family trusted me implicitly and had no other good options so they started the real food way of eating and whole food supplements.

Here's what happened in Davis' own words:

"Now 3 months later, my heart function is within 5 percent of normal and I don't need a pacemaker. I can now work like I used to and even started an exercise program at the YMCA. I feel better than I have in years. As an added benefit, I am losing weight and got off all those drugs. My cardiologist couldn't believe how much better my tests were and said he had never seen or heard of this happening."

That's the potential power of natural care.

The healthiest patients I see are those who take no prescription medication. Here's an example. "Don and Mildred," a couple in their early 90s, looked like vibrantly healthy people in their late sixties. They had very few symptoms, wore big smiles and, after 65 years of marriage, still held hands like two love birds.

I asked when their last medical exam was. They looked at each other and started laughing. "We haven't seen a medical doctor since our last one died," one said. "How long ago was that?" I asked. "1958!"

To be clear, I'm not recommending this for anyone. I believe we each should have an excellent integrative medical doctor as well as a natural health care team. Both are important when used judiciously.

As I questioned this couple further, I discovered that they had never been inside a fast-food restaurant. They did yoga and walked each day and grew a big garden. They loved each other and their many family and friends. Their lives reflected the quality of their self-care.

Don died several years later when he fell on the ice and hit his head. Mildred passed on peacefully in her sleep just a few months later. That's radiant wellness.

If you want that for you and your loved ones, choose natural health care approaches whenever possible. Lovingly care for your body and educate yourself about self-care strategies. Recognize that your body has an inner wisdom and *work with it* to reach and maintain well being. By doing so, you may prevent serious health problems that require crisis care treatment.

Achieving total wellness is not that difficult. As Norman Cousins, author of *Anatomy of an Illness,* stated, "Plainly, the American people need to be reeducated about their health. They need to know that they are the possessors of a remarkably robust mechanism. They need to be deintimidated about disease... We are much stronger than we think. Much stronger."

Why Natural Care?

As we've discussed, natural healing approaches are almost always very safe, affordable and effective. That's why, whenever possible, it's wise to consider natural health care before drugs and surgery.

I'm well aware of the importance of orthodox medical care. I worked in hospitals for six years and have had numerous family and friends in the medical field. Medical care is very important for *crisis or emergency care,* for example, a broken bone, ruptured appendix, severe trauma, or potentially fatal illness. Many very intelligent and committed caregivers provide medical and surgical treatment. I wouldn't want to practice natural health care without that backup.

For example, my brother's neighbor nearly had his arm cut off. Even though it was dangling by just a few nerves and blood vessels, medical specialists helped him regain full use of his arm. His father-in-law had a ruptured abdominal aortic aneurysm and, thanks to emergency treatment, lived to see his grandchildren grow up and two great-grandchildren born. My dad developed lung cancer. Half of one lung was removed and he lived another 12 years to 80 years of age.

All of this is very impressive.

However, drug and surgical treatments have little to offer for many common ailments. What's worse, the side effects of those approaches can *be worse than the original symptoms.*

That's not just my opinion. Many medical doctors and natural health experts have come to the same conclusion.

Andrew Weil MD, author of *Spontaneous Healing* and *8 Weeks to Optimum Health,* recognizes the importance of medical treatment for emergency situations, but states: "Although allopaths (orthodox medical doctors) give lip service to the concept of preventive medicine, for practical purposes they are unable to prevent most of the diseases that disable and kill people today."

As mentioned, drugs and surgery often interfere with normal body functioning, have serious potential side effects and are expensive. In addition, these invasive approaches don't *address the underlying* causes of disease.

Here's an example of the last point. Thirty-year-old Frank consulted me for his headaches and neck pain. During the history, I found he had been on blood pressure medication for two years. His medical doctor put him on those drugs *after just one* high blood pressure reading.

Frank was moderately overweight, didn't exercise, ate a poor diet, smoked cigarettes, and was very stressed after a recent divorce. His doctor did not ask about any of these details, but just put him on medication. That's a classic example of misusing prescription medication and not addressing the underlying causes of the problem.

Historically, about 95 percent of health problems in China have been addressed with natural methods—primarily acupuncture, nutrition and herbs, spinal manipulation, and massage. Only about 5 percent required drugs and surgery. In the U.S., it has been the reverse, but that trend is changing and for good reason.

Deepak Chopra MD states, "About 80 percent of all the drugs that we use in western medicine are `optional' or of marginal benefit, which means that if we didn't use them, it wouldn't make a bit of difference to the person except save money and prevent side effects

...When we use drugs as indiscriminately as we do currently, we see some problems."

Major problems. In fact, orthodox approaches can make a person *much worse or dead* due to side effects, errors and complications. I've seen this many times and numerous medical studies document the severity of this issue. A large number of my patients have suffered new and serious problems after surgery or taking medications for relatively minor ailments.

An attempt by the medical system to put everyone into a contrived norm is part of the problem. Remember the 90-something patient named Mildred? Her blood pressure was 180/100, had been for many years, and she felt great. Since I was her only doctor, I encouraged her to see a medical doctor about her blood pressure. He put her on blood pressure lowering medications and, within a few weeks, her blood pressure was closer to normal. But Mildred felt horrible.

"I feel weak, dizzy and tired all the time," she said. "I'd rather feel great and die sooner than take that medication, feel horrible, and live longer." I couldn't argue with her logic. She quit the drugs, her blood pressure elevated, and she felt and functioned great.

Years later, I read that the "normal" 120/80 blood pressure value was created by a medical study involving a few dozen people. That was their average blood pressure, and that's been the norm ever since. But is that blood pressure the optimal reading for everyone?

More recent medical studies have recommended changing the norm for blood pressure over age 60 (if no diabetes or kidney disease) to 150/90. But many medical doctors don't know about those findings. So many elderly people are given dangerous drugs to lower their blood pressure to unhealthfully low levels that aren't supported some studies.

Same song, different verse with total cholesterol values. For decades, 260 mg/DL or below was considered normal. Then that number was changed to 240, then 220, then 200 and now many millions of Americans supposedly needed medication. Many astute observers, including medical doctors, have noted that these lab values changed after several large pharmaceutical companies developed new cholesterol lowering drugs.

Probably just a coincidence.

I've had numerous patients who were put on bladder medications when their only symptom was getting up to urinate once during the night. Somewhere in antiquity, some genius – probably the same guy who said it's normal to have one bowel movement per week – said you shouldn't have to get up at night to urinate.

Let's examine that one for a moment with a little common sense. Do you go eight hours through the day without urinating? I hope not. Then why should you be able to do so during the night? If you drink sufficient water, you should have to urinate once during the night.

But I digress. We were talking about medical treatment causing new or worse symptoms than the original problem.

John McDougall MD, author of *The McDougall Plan,* states: "Most medical treatments for long-standing diseases can honestly be called patch jobs and temporary fixes ...Simple, sensible, safe, self-help approaches based upon a healthy diet and an equally healthy lifestyle are almost never mentioned by doctors. Instead, almost routinely, life-threatening drugs and dangerous surgeries are prescribed as if no other avenue of treatment were available."

Other serious side effects from commonly used medications:

- ***antiinflammatory drugs:*** *heart attacks, stroke, and gastrointestinal bleeding*
- ***antiosteoporosis drugs:*** *brittle bones and osteonecrosis (bone death)*
- ***pain killers (including over-the-counter ones):*** *liver, kidney, and stomach disease*
- ***antidepressants:*** *increased homicide and suicide*
- ***ADD/ADHD drugs:*** *heart attack, stroke and death.*

People who watch a lot of TV may be overly influenced by drug commercials. *Ask your doctor...*

Abuse of prescription pain killing drugs is another downside of conventional medical treatment. Many people have died from drug addictions. Even more have battled through the nightmare that began because of drugs prescribed for physical or emotional pain that might have been helped by natural health care. But insurance often doesn't cover natural care so people are economically forced to get the drugs and entire families can be devastated.

In the worse case scenario, *medical treatment for common ailments causes death.* That fact has been well documented and makes a convincing case for natural healing approaches whenever possible. A Yale-New Haven Hospital Study in the 1980s estimated that 100,000 Americans die annually from prescription drug reactions. In the 1990s, a *USA Today* article put this figure at 180,000 deaths, while Ralph Nader's estimate was 300,000.

Most recently, the prestigious *New England Journal of Medicine* (JAMA) reported that over 750,000 Americans die *each year* from prescription drug reactions, hospital borne infections, complications from unnecessary surgeries, and outright mistakes. Mark Hyman MD, discusses these figures in his book *The Five Forces of Wellness.*

Other excellent books that discuss the serious dangers of orthodox medical treatment include *What Doctors Don't Tell You* by Lynne McTaggart, and *Death by Medicine* by Gary Null PhD, Martin Feldman MD, Debora Rasio MD, and Carolyn Dean MD, ND.

In addition to the cost in human lives and suffering, the monetary cost of medical mistakes and side effects are in the hundreds of billions of dollars per year. But don't hold your breath waiting for the medical system to police itself. Nearly three trillion dollars per year can cause some people to justify needlessly invasive and harmful treatments.

Make no mistake about it. The disease care industry – hospitals, pharmaceutical companies, medical schools, medical device makers, and insurance companies – is big, big business. Most doctors, nurses, and other caregivers are very caring and dedicated. But a number of emerging studies clearly show that *decision makers* don't always have the patient's welfare as their number one priority.

For example, studies reported in JAMA show that two-thirds of teachers surveyed at U.S. medical schools and teaching hospitals have financial ties to pharmaceutical companies and medical device makers. Their biases for drug and surgical approaches is passed on to medical students even though safe and effective natural treatments exist.

Tim suffered with nearly constant and significant chest pain for ten years. Medical treatment during that time consisted of five stents and numerous drugs that were all paid for by his insurance company. When he came to our office, I recommended chiropractic adjustments of the sternum and ribs. (Misalignment of those bones can cause chest pain, shortness of breath, irregular heart rhythm, and anxiety/panic feelings.)

Tim's insurance didn't cover chiropractic so I adjusted these areas at no extra charge. After just four treatments, his chest pain was gone and didn't come back. Months later, he said, "Do you mean I had all those stents put in and took all those drugs for nothing?" Maybe.

Isn't it about time for people to wake up to these issues and take more responsibility for their health? How many more people must suffer and die before we learn that mega-businesses can't be trusted to know what is best?

Recently released court documents showed that one large pharmaceutical company *paid ghostwriters* to create 26 scientific papers backing the use of hormone replacement therapy in women. This and similar pending cases point to *hidden industry influence* on medical research. Sales of these drugs soared until a large government study was halted because of increased heart disease, breast cancer, stroke, and dementia among women taking them.

Patients trust their medical doctors to give the best treatment. Many doctors are caring and intelligent, but they are also influenced by multi-trillion dollar per year businesses. It's not a good system. I warn my patients *to beware* that huge profit margins in medical care can influence their recommendations.

I spoke with a retired hospital CEO about the power of natural health care and self-care practices such as eating a chemical-free whole food diet. "When do you think the medical profession will wake up and start recommending that?" I asked him. He didn't hesitate, "Never. There's no money in it. Why would they teach about natural treatment when they can do a heart bypass for $100,000?"

Over the years, I have had a number of friends and family in the medical profession. Those who contract with hospitals tell me that *they get yelled at* if they take too much time with patients and try to educate them.

Urgent care facility managers want the doctors to quickly write prescriptions, then move on to the next patient. These doctors gain or lose staff privileges based on whether they refer more or fewer *big money cases:* expensive diagnostic tests, surgical cases, and patients who need hospitalized.

Not a good system when a patient's health and life are at stake.

To be fair, the medical-pharmacological industry is not solely at fault. They provide what many people want: *supposedly quick fixes* versus changing their lifestyles and being patient for the body to heal itself.

In my experience, only 1 out of 10 people take control of their health and their lives. People often don't do what it takes to enjoy high levels of health and prevent problems. They wait until they're in a crisis and then expect doctors to bail them out.

Choosing this *disease care option* has disastrous consequences. I encourage you to take self-responsibility and choose natural health care for yourself and your loved ones whenever possible.

Common Natural Health Care Approaches

Some people don't know about natural health care and subsequently can't enjoy the potential benefits. Others may try these approaches for a while, but give up when instant results aren't forthcoming. Natural healing can take time, especially for chronic cases.

Here's an overview in alphabetical order of the most common natural care treatments. Additional resources are listed and an internet search will provide more information. I discuss several approaches in further detail since they are so foundational for radiant wellness.

Acupuncture

This millennia-old healing approach uses very tiny needles inserted into specific points on the skin, *meridian points* that correspond to certain organs and muscles. Acupuncture helps strengthen and balance the flow of energy or *chi.* In the Orient, acupuncture has long been used as a primary healing modality and even anesthesia during major surgery. The safety and effectiveness of this approach are well documented.

In the U.S., acupuncture can be performed by specially trained health care providers: LAc (licensed acupuncturist), OMD (oriental medical doctor), and DAC (doctor of acupuncture). Chiropractic, medical, and osteopathic physicians may practice acupuncture after additional training. However, that instruction is a fraction of what is required for a LAc, OMD, and DAC.

When healthy, I get at least quarterly acupuncture sessions to ensure optimal balance and movement of energy to all parts of my body. If I develop any symptoms, acupuncture is an important part of my therapeutic program.

For example, during a time of extreme stress, I developed a tremor of my right thumb. My integrative medical doctor administered several acupuncture treatments and the shaking went away. Who knows what might have developed had I not quickly and effectively addressed the source of the problem.

For additional information, visit ***nccaom.org*** (National Certification Commission for Acupuncture and Oriental Medicine); ***acaom.com*** (Accreditation Commission for Acupuncture and Oriental Medicine); and ***www.nccam.nih.gov/health/acupuncture*** (National Center for Complementary and Alternative Medicine as part of NIH.)

Alternative Medicine

An increasing number of allopathic (MD) and osteopathic (DO) physicians are using alternative medical approaches. Synonyms for alternative include complementary, integrative, functional and pro-medicine. These doctors understand the downsides of drug and surgical approaches and use more conservative measures whenever possible. I've learned much about this field from Andrew Weil MD, Dean Ornish MD, Julian Whitaker MD, Joseph Mercola DO, Mark Hyman MD, and Allan Magaziner DO.

Alternative medical doctors may use acupuncture, spinal and cranial manipulation, chelation therapy, dietary modification, nutritional supplements, hyperbaric oxygen, homeopathy, heavy metal removal, light therapy, nutritional IV therapy, lifestyle counseling and other more natural modalities.

In general, they use *pro-life* methods that *work with* the wisdom of the body, for example, recommending probiotics instead of or after antibiotics. The goal of alternative medical approaches is to assist the body in regaining wellness instead of fighting a war against disease and viewing the body as a passive and ignorant battlefield. *This is a crucial distinction.*

Select an integrative medical doctor who uses natural health care whenever possible and can identify severe health problems that require medication or surgery. Doctors who practice this way can be located via ACAM (American College of Advanced Medicine), AHMA (American Holistic Medical Association), and ABHM (American Board of Holistic Medicine.)

Body Awareness Movements

This term describes techniques that increase overall wellness by movement and positions of the body. These include tai chi, qi gong, yoga, and other integrated techniques. Various forms of dance such as Nia enhance wellness via movement, breathing, and social connections. Cross-cultural dances and body prayers such as those taught by Neil Douglas-Klotz PhD provide holistic benefits.

Chiropractic Care

Ideally, a doctor of chiropractic (DC) *makes specific spinal adjustments,* not gross manipulations, to correct vertebral subluxation. A *subluxation* is a minor misalignment and/or fixation of vertebrae that exerts slight pressure on the spinal cord and nerves. Chiropractic care can relieve pain, prevent arthritic degeneration, and assist a healthy nervous system.

A normal nerve supply is required for the brain to communicate with all body parts and vice-versa. Much chiropractic, allopathic, and osteopathic research has verified that abnormal nerve function caused by subluxation can result in many different symptoms and diseases.

Babies should have their spinal, cranial, and skeletal bones checked since the birth process can be traumatic. All people should be evaluated regularly throughout life, especially after any trauma and if there are health problems.

Counseling

As discussed, psychological and/or pastoral counseling is important for reestablishing emotional and spiritual balance. I favor *outcome-oriented approaches* that are time limited versus involving years of ongoing analysis. Keep this natural treatment approach in mind, especially when you are dealing with lots of stress or feel that you lack clarity to make important decisions.

Cranial Adjustments

Skillful and gentle adjustments of bones of the skull can restore normal position and micro-movement. This can be done by a specially trained physician or craniosacral therapist.

Recently a two-year-old boy suffering with 'congenital torticollis' was brought to my office. That big diagnostic term means Ely's head had been bent to one side since he was born. His condition was unchanged despite seeing pediatric orthopedists at a children's hospital and wearing a specially made brace.

I evaluated him and gently adjusted three cranial bones that were stuck and/or slightly out of alignment. Several days later, he and his mother returned for a follow-up visit. "His neck has been totally normal since we left your office," the mother beamed. Just a few more visits were required to *correct* the misalignments and he has been fine ever since.

Cranial bones can become slightly misaligned or fixated after the birth process or any trauma to the head. The skull bones house the brain, blood vessels, and cranial nerves so minor misalignments can cause major problems. Cranial adjusting has been successful in helping a wide variety of physical and mental disorders. Much research has documented the safety and effectiveness of cranial adjusting.

For more information, read books by or visit websites of: Tedd Koren, DC (***KorenSpecificTechnique.com***) Sacro Occipital Research Society International (***Sorsi.com***), and John Upledger, DO (***Upledger.com***)

As with the spine, people of all ages should have their cranial bones evaluated. Why wait until there is a problem?

Energy Healing

Numerous energy healing and balancing techniques can remove tension and increase harmony of body functions. These approaches make sense since we are, from a quantum level, beings of energy.

Energy flows that are blocked and imbalanced may be improved by: Touch for Health, Therapeutic Touch, Polarity Therapy, Body Talk, Reiki, and Network Chiropractic.

Essential Oil Therapy

This healing approach is also known as "Aromatherapy" but that's a misnomer since its effectiveness is not due to fragrance. The leaves, stems, roots and seeds of many plants can have powerful healing effects. I especially recommend essential oil therapy products formulated by Andy Lee RN, LAc, CCA. (***AndyLLee.com***) For example, her *Joyful Body blend* combines six oils to decrease pain, inflammation, and spasm. We use this, Glory Be, CBD, and other of her products at my office.

Other examples of oils include: peppermint oil (for GI upset); lavender oil for sunburn, bug bites and emotional calming; tea tree oil for infections, acne, and toothache. For more information about this amazing healing approach, read *The Complete Book of Essential Oils and Aromatherapy* by Valerie Ann Worwood.

Holistic Dentistry

Holistic dentists may use biocompatible fillings, mercury free procedures, nutrition for the oral cavity, and other natural methods. These practitioners also are aware of *cavitations,* focal points of infection that can occur around the base of a tooth, especially after a root canal.

I had my mercury fillings taken out many years ago and recommend that my patients refrain from getting mercury fillings. People with significant physical and mental symptoms that have not responded to other healing methods may want to consider mercury removal. For more information about this important topic, visit ***iaomt.org*** (International Academy of Oral Medicine and Toxicology) and ***holisticdental.org*** (Holistic Dental Association).

Hypnotherapy

Hypnotherapy has been widely and safely used for centuries to deeply relax the body so the brain is more open to positive suggestions.

It can be used for smoking cessation, weight loss, pain relief, stress management, and overcoming phobias. Hypnotherapy also can help eliminate limiting beliefs that may interfere with one's life.

I use hypnosis during several psycho-spiritual integration techniques when working with groups. I personally receive quarterly hypnosis sessions for stress management, clarity, and focus.

To find a reputable hypno-therapist in your area, contact ***ngh.net*** (National Guild of Hypnotists) or ***imdha.com*** (International Medical and Dental Hypnosis Association).

Massage

Massage assists emotional and physical well being. In Europe, doctors are as likely to prescribe a series of massage as they are tranquilizers. The many benefits of massage include: relief of stress, tension and pain; increased circulation, flexibility and relaxation; and a calmer and more creative state of mind.

Different forms of massage may be more effective for your needs. For example, Rolfing addresses myofascial tension, Swedish massage is for deeper muscle work, and hot stone and oil therapies provide profound relaxation. Reflexology is a massage system for the feet that addresses structural fixations, reflex response, and energy balancing.

Nutrition-Based Healing Approaches

Knowledgeable health care practitioners using these methods will recommend a real food way of eating, whole food supplements, herbs and specific regimens to restore wellness. In addition to physicians and acupuncturists, this method may be used by naturopathic doctors (ND) and holistically trained registered or licensed dieticians (RD or LD).

I'll discuss this approach more fully later in the chapter.

Other Modalities

These include therapies using sound, color, aromatherapy and energetic crystals. Sound therapy can be provided by tuning forks, toning and CDs with specific tones. Color therapy uses lights of different colors. Certain fragrances can impact the body and brain in healing ways.

High tech combinations of these can be especially effective for a number of emotional and physical ailments. I send some of my tough cases to other highly trained health care professionals who use these approaches. The future of health care will, no doubt, see more and more use of these powerful modalities.

Physical Therapy

A LPT or DPT provides noninvasive care for joints, muscles, tendons, ligaments, and discs. They employ a combination of stretching, strengthening, education, and various modalities to restore normal function and range of motion to these areas.

Having reviewed a number of natural health care approaches, I will discuss three that I consider especially useful in more detail.

Acupuncture

Acupuncture has its roots in traditional Chinese medicine (TCM).

TCM theory states that your body, like everything else in nature, is able to function at its best when in a state of *balance.* Many factors

– physical and emotional trauma, inadequate rest and improper diet, for example—can push your body toward *imbalance.*

Imbalances can cause your body to feel sick, experience pain, or function improperly. Acupuncture works by helping the body move toward a *balanced state.* Small needles act like *antennae* that alert your awareness to where imbalances are so it can begin to heal.

Two ways to explain acupuncture: a Traditional Chinese Medicine (TCM) or western medicine perspective. In the TCM model, pathways called meridians run along the surface of your body. Circulating in these pathways is qi or chi (pronounced "chee"), an invisible energy that gives you life and keeps you healthy.

When qi moves freely throughout the meridians and your body is in balance, you are healthy. However, when qi gets low or stagnated, the natural balance of your body is disrupted and illness can result. Causes of *imbalanced chi* include too injury, strong emotions, inactivity, poor nutrition, heredity, too little or too much sleep, etc.

In western medicine terms, the effects of acupuncture are called the "mechanism of action." Many studies have shown that acupuncture promotes circulation, reduces inflammation, releases pain-inhibiting endorphins, regulates endocrine function, and increases immune function.

Acupuncture has been used to treat hundreds of different ailments for at least 2500 years. The World Health Organization and National Institutes of Health endorse acupuncture for the treatment of over 140 conditions, including muscle and joint pain, diarrhea, insomnia, TMJ, joint strain/sprain, sciatica, low energy, cataracts, stroke, infertility, abdominal pain, anxiety, allergies, headache, chemo side effects, carpal tunnel, rheumatoid arthritis, painful menstrual cycle, constipation, depression, asthma, hypertension, fibromyalgia, addictions, tennis elbow, erectile dysfunction, facial pain, labor induction, tooth pain, Bell's palsy, gall bladder stones, earache, fasciitis, gouty arthritis, obesity, PMS, rectal itching, urinary tract infections, kidney stones, IBS, morning sickness, gastritis, ulcers, labor induction, low back pain, stiff neck, ulcerative colitis, diabetes, lactation deficiency, neuralgia and many more.

The vast majority of patients experience no pain during treatment. In fact, most find that acupuncture is a very relaxing experience. When needles are inserted, you may feel an energetic sensation such as slight tingling or heaviness in the area. This is called "de qi" or "the arrival of qi."

All acupuncture needles are approved by the FDA and are sterile, single-use disposables. The needles vary in length and width, but most are no thicker than a human hair. They are also very flexible like a cat's whisker. There are *needle-free options* for those who are afraid of even very thin and short needles. These include Chinese massage (tui na), acupressure, heat therapy, cupping, and scraping (gua sha.)

There are very few, if any, negative side effects after a treatment. Rarely, a patient may experience slight bruising around the insertion site; inform your acupuncturist before beginning treatment if you take aspirin or other blood-thinning medication. Rarely, patients feel slightly dizzy or nauseous after a treatment. This is generally due to receiving acupuncture on an empty stomach.

Acupuncture does not interact or interfere with any medication. However, patients may find that, as their health improves, they no longer require the same medication dose. It is important that you work with your doctor to adjust your prescriptions accordingly.

As a youth, I saw a TV show about acupuncture being used in China for anesthesia during surgery. *Wide-awake* people were talking calmly while surgeons operated inside their thoracic or abdominal cavities! I knew then that acupuncture was amazing and it is. I highly recommend that you and your loved ones use it for prevention and therapeutic purposes.

Chiropractic

Minor misalignment of the spine, skull and skeletal bones can cause *major* health problems. Chiropractors adjust misalignments of these bones to prevent or treat symptoms and disease.

Chiropractic is gaining wider acceptance because it fills a *vital niche* in health care. Chiropractic physicians who use specific and advanced methods do much more than relieve back pain; *they are nerve and spinal specialists.*

One definition of chiropractic is, "A health science built on the premise that within man there is an intelligent, constructive force operating through clearly defined channels. It is this *life force* that generates, develops and maintains our bodies from conception to grave."

A misaligned and fixated bone of the spine is called a *vertebral subluxation complex* (VSC) because it can trigger an array of related problems. When bones are out of alignment, surrounding tissues—cartilage, muscles, ligaments, tendons, nerves and blood vessels—can be adversely affected.

Subluxations can be caused by *trauma* during the birth process, especially with prolonged or difficult labor and abnormal presentation. The use of forceps, vacuum delivery or caesareans may increase the incidence of spinal misalignment.

Other causes of misaligned spinal bones include falls, sports injuries, auto accidents, work injuries and repetitive motions. Subluxation can also be caused by poor waking posture, abnormal sleep posture, improper pillow and mattress, poor general health, and muscle weakness and imbalance.

Symptoms of nerve pressure include pain, numbness, tingling, burning, hot or cold sensations, itching, aching, cramping, weakness or other abnormal sensations. However, subluxation can also be a silent process, like high blood pressure, so ***you can't rely on symptoms*** to know whether vertebral subluxation exists.

Disorders caused by nerve pressure are divided into two categories: *neuro-musculo-skeletal* (NMS) and *visceral.*

Many people associate chiropractic with relief of NMS problems because it can work wonders with back and neck pain and radiation of nerve pressure symptoms into the head, arms, and legs. Related symptoms include muscle weakness, restless and cramping legs, muscle twitches and tremors.

These may not sound like a big deal on paper, but they were to the people we helped who suffered with Tourette Syndrome, Multiple Sclerosis, seizures, and other NMS ailments. It's important to address these serious conditions as early as possible since, in my experience, natural care usually doesn't help once patients are wheelchair bound.

I could fill a book with successful NMS cases but will share just three:

1. *Robert was a surgeon who came to me for treatment of severe chronic pain. Fifteen years of using pain medication resulted in drug addiction. He lost his license to practice, was depressed, and his life was falling apart. His symptoms were completely gone after six months of chiropractic care and his license was eventually reinstated.*
2. *Mae suffered with* ***severe migraine headaches every day for forty-five years.*** *She had been to eleven medical headache clinics around the country and was told she had three types of rare incurable migraines. Her headaches went away completely after three spinal adjustments.*
3. *Sarah was brought in because she couldn't walk normally, climb stairs, and or ride a bike. Medical specialists thought she had either muscular dystrophy or multiple sclerosis. After a few months of spinal adjustments, Sarah was totally normal and a year later made the junior high cheerleading squad. Twenty years later, she is very healthy, but her legs "feel funny" if she goes more than a few months between adjustments.*

Organic or visceral conditions are also often helped by specific and corrective chiropractic adjustments. *We've assisted* (I say 'assisted' because the body does the healing) significant improvement or total cures with the following: migraines, visual disturbances, loss of smell, dizziness, hearing loss, tinnitus, sinus conditions, allergies, asthma, high blood pressure, rapid or irregular heart beat, recurrent infections, indigestion, ulcers, constipation, diarrhea, colitis, Crohn's disease, bloating and excess gas, irritable bowel syndrome, sexual dysfunction, anxiety, nervousness, depression, infertility, erectile dysfunction, insomnia, urinary urgency or difficulty, bedwetting, hemorrhoids, and painful or irregular menstrual cycles.

A few actual cases of visceral improvement:

1. *Bruce, a nine-year-old boy, wet the bed every night. In addition, he often had bowel movements without any warning. Both symptoms were, needless to say, terribly embarrassing and went away after receiving spinal adjustments.*
2. *Susan, a forty-year old, suffered with severe menstrual cramps, excessive bleeding, and irregular cycles. Her upper lumbar vertebrae, where nerves supply the reproductive system, were misaligned. To her astonishment, her periods became totally normal within two months of chiropractic care.*
3. *Don, the administrator of a large hospital in another city, came to me because he didn't want anyone to know he was going to a DC. He reported chronic and severe backache and headaches. But his lateral neck was* ***curved the wrong way*** *and the arthritic pattern suggested it had been that way for about 20 years.*

I told him, "You're telling me about your back pain and headaches but, if you're like most patients with a reversed neck, you're also experiencing insomnia, depression, fatigue and anxiety. You're wondering how your days have become so dreary and lifeless." As I told him this, a tear ran down his cheek and his wife said, "You just described him exactly for the last three years." After corrective spinal care, he reported complete improvement of all symptoms and a dramatic increase in energy.

These organic improvements are possible because adjustments allow normal function of the autonomic nervous system, the nerves that connect the brain with every organ in the body. Nutritional approaches are often needed to help difficult problems.

It is important to select *an outstanding chiropractor* who uses advanced methods and provides *spinal correction,* not just relief care.

Find a DC who takes spinal x-rays, reevaluates improvement, and uses *full-spine adjusting.*

In summary, remember that spinal vertebrae, can become stuck and/or misaligned and put slight pressure on nerves, blood vessels, and other soft tissues. This, in turn, can cause many common symptoms and diseases. Fortunately, subluxations can be treated painlessly, safely and relatively inexpensively.

If you or your loved ones are suffering and you think you've tried every possible treatment, you haven't tried everything unless you've tried specific chiropractic.

For additional information, read: *Chiropractors—Do They Help?* by Kelner, Hall, and Coulter; *The Confusion About Chiropractors* by Richard E. DeRoeck DC; *Chiropractic and Spinal Research* by Tedd Koren DC; *So You're Thinking of Going to a Chiropractor* by Robert Dryburgh DC; and *Chiropractic First* by Terry Rondberg DC.

Nutrition-Based Health Care

It's quite a challenge to determine exactly what is *at the core* of a person's health problems. There are many possible causes that can lead to common physical and mental ailments.

I've used several methods for detecting and correcting *interferences* (too *many* stressors) and deficiencies (too *few* nutrients). I now recommend Nutrition Response Testing (***unsinc.info***) and Applied Kinesiology (***icakusa.com***).

We've helped many *people heal themselves* of the following health conditions: depression, fatigue, tremors, overweight, anxiety, insomnia, constipation, diarrhea, allergies, sinus drainage and congestion, cold hands and feet, memory loss, facial twitches, rectal itching and burning, indigestion, night sweats, hot flashes, tender breasts, mood swings, muscle cramps, sweet cravings, bad breath, brain fog, shakiness, skin rash, acne, irritability, dizziness, nervousness, panic attacks, frequent colds and flu, visual disturbances, sneezing attacks, joint pain, hair loss, urinary frequency/urgency/incontinence, high blood pressure, high blood sugar, high cholesterol, imbalance/vertigo, heart arrhythmias, and ridged and split nails.

Named diseases or syndromes that have improved significantly or totally include: multiple sclerosis, crohn's disease, lyme's disease, irritable bowel syndrome, cardiomyopathy, diabetes, neuropathy, lupus and other autoimmune disorders, ADD/ADHD, autism, raynaud's disease, asthma, GERD, chronic fatigue syndrome, ulcer, gall bladder disease, colitis, erectile dysfunction, benign prostatic hypertrophy, alzheimer disease, psoriasis, eczema, liver disease, and more.

I do not capitalize these symptoms and diseases because they do not really exist as distinct entities. They are *expressions of imbalance* that can be addressed. The body can't speak English or any other language, so it speaks in symptoms.

I'm amazed at how *seemingly incurable* cases improve over time with nutrition-based healing approaches. This has revolutionized how I look at the human body and what it is capable of. If caught early enough, the great majority of diseases, syndromes and symptoms clear up nicely with this approach. I'll mention several common areas of suffering and associated key factors.

1. ***Perimenopausal symptoms*** *that occur before, during and after the menopause can include hot flashes, night sweats, mood swings, weight gain, sleep disturbance, fatigue, decreased libido, vaginal dryness, brittle nails, hair loss, dry skin and bone loss. When the ovaries decrease functioning, the adrenal glands are supposed to provide backup by producing small amounts of female hormones.*

   However, if one or more parts of the endocrine system – pituitary, thyroid, hypothalamus, and adrenals especially – are weak or imbalanced, the symptoms above occur. It's the difference between menopause being like a bump in the road versus a rollercoaster ride from hell. Fortunately, the above symptoms usually respond well to holistic and nutrition-based health care.

2. ***Mental symptoms** include depression, nervousness, panic attacks, ADD/ADHD, obsessive-compulsive disorder, memory loss and loss of mental concentration. These often respond very well when patients follow a program of eating real food and providing the brain and hormonal organs with necessary nutrients.*

3. ***Chronic sinus conditions** such as drainage, congestion, recurrent infection, sneezing and coughing are so common. The sinuses are a perfect breeding grounds for microorganism growth. A high sugar and carbohydrate diet assists* **exponential growth** *of viruses, bacteria and yeast/fungus. Nutrition-based healing boost the immune system and gets the number and types of microorganisms under control.*

4. ***Digestive system symptoms** including constipation, diarrhea, excess gas, and more affect many people. The most common causes are poor diet, insufficient gastric acid and digestive enzymes, offending foods, antibiotic use, and overgrowth of harmful microorganisms. These factors can almost always be relieved or completely cured.*

———◆———

Nutrition-based healthcare programs use subtle muscle testing to get a *binary indicator*—'yes or no' answer—from the body. This feedback allows health practitioners to accurately and safely analyze if any *neurological interference, stressor or nutritional deficiency* is causing abnormal body function.

These three *core causes* are often at the root of many common physical and mental symptoms and include:

A. Neurological Interference:

***1. ANS Imbalance or blocking:** your body is not "open" to healing as it should be*

2. Switching: *your body has a back and forth or opposite reaction to treatment instead of steady improvement*

B. Stressors:

1. Offending Foods: *foods such as wheat, sugar, dairy, soy, etc. that can trigger many different symptoms*

2. Immune Challenges: *an overgrowth of viruses, bacteria, yeast/fungus or parasites*

3. Electro-Magnetic Fields: *'dirty energy' from electronic devices that can negatively impact the body*

4. Excess Chemicals: *due to the 2,000 or more chemicals we are exposed to daily*

5. Toxic Metals: *aluminum, arsenic, mercury, lead, etc.*

6. Scars: *from surgery, cuts, body piercings, tattoos, stretch marks and injections/IV sites*

C. Nutritional Deficiencies:

1. Deficiencies of minerals, *vitamins, cofactors, essential fatty acids, and other vital nutrients*

2. Lack of digestive enzymes, *hydrochloric acid, good bacteria and yeast*

3. Insufficient nutrients, *but excessive trans fats, omega 6 oils, pesticides, herbicides, genetically modified (GMO) seeds, etc.*

Natural Care for Children

Natural health care is especially important for children. Fortunately, they usually respond quickly and completely to natural healing methods.

Five-month-old Tiffany was brought to my office by her mother and grandmother. Tiffany had suffered with *severe colic* her entire life and cried 90 percent of the time night and day. The family first took her to a pediatrician who prescribed medications for indigestion and for pain.

While taking the history, I discovered the mother didn't breastfeed and Tiffany had eaten only soy-based formulas and cow's milk. After evaluating her, I found that this little one was allergic to cow's milk and soy products. The medical doctors never asked about her diet. Her crying was the only way she could communicate that what she was being fed did not agree with her system.

I also found a need for supplemental digestive enzymes and a whole food supplement to soothe the inflamed stomach and esophageal tissues. I instructed the family to feed her rice and almond milk along with homemade baby food from fresh healthy ingredients.

In one week, Tiffany was 75 percent better. In two weeks, she was 100 percent better. Several months later, she is totally fine and needs no supplements. Case solved safely, inexpensively and without drugs that may have caused future problems.

Natural healing methods often work wonderfully with children. I want you to know about conservative treatment options for the little ones in your life.

Here are a few topics that pertain to children's needs. Remember the 3 L's when having a baby: Leboyer, La Leche and Lamaze. These three approaches to childbirth and infant care provide an outstanding start.

The Leboyer method stresses a drug-free and gentle teamwork approach to birthing. French obstetrician Dr. Frederick Leboyer described this technique in his book *Birth without Violence.* Dim lights, peaceful music, a warm bath, and skin-on-skin contact provide the most reassuring environment just after birth. We used these approaches with the births of our daughters and the hospital staff said they had never seen such *alert and relaxed* babies.

The topic of breastfeeding was discussed in the Diet chapter but it's so important that it bears repeating. Breastfeeding—as taught by *the La Leche League* and the book *The Womanly Art of Breastfeeding*—gives a newborn ideal nutritional and psychological support.

Our daughters were breastfed exclusively until they were ready for solid foods. They continued to nurse less and less until the age two when they weaned themselves. Breastfeeding is a free, easy, and vastly superior approach to infant nutrition.

It's sad that many mothers do not use this *naturally right* approach. Cow's milk, soy milk, and commercially prepared formulas are poor –and possibly even dangerous – substitutes for the real thing. Food allergies are just one negative result of a baby consuming any food except breast milk.

The *Lamaze method* trains mothers to give birth with no or minimal use of drugs that can affect the baby.

Holistically oriented nurse midwives and OB nurse practitioners can greatly enhance every aspect of the birth process including optimal prenatal and postnatal care for mother and child.

Another critical natural health care topic for children is the issue of *vaccinations*. Questioning vaccination programs may sound absurd to those who trust authority without question. After all, pediatricians, health departments, pharmacies, billboards and newspaper ads widely recommend them. Right?

More and more doctors and parents are questioning the wisdom of so many vaccinations, nearly 80 recommended by school age, or any at all. Growing evidence shows how common and serious adverse reactions are.

In our practice, several mothers have brought in their little ones who suffer from autism and other neurological disorders. These mothers, who know better than anyone, swear that their children were perfectly normal until just after vaccinations were given.

Some natural health experts, for example, Andrew Weil MD, believe that the risks for most vaccinations are acceptable when compared to the benefits. He doesn't recommend the chicken pox vaccine and believes the hepatitis B vaccine should only be used for atrisk populations.

Many other MDs, DOs and DCs believe that, when optimal prenatal and postnatal care is given, the risks of vaccinations are not worth the benefits. However, if substandard health care conditions exist – in impoverished areas with poor sanitation, for example – the benefits may be worth the risks.

This is a complex and emotionally charged topic; I encourage readers to educate themselves about it. The lives and health of the children in your life depend on it.

I believe that, in the future, people will look at current practices such as routine vaccinations and ask, "Do you mean that back then parents really had their children injected with unproven and dangerous drugs? Why didn't the government and health care providers warn them about the dangers?" Great questions. The good news is that, for you and the little ones if your life, the future can be now.

Pro-vaccination arguments are well known since shots are widely administered by orthodox health systems and pharmacies. *Concerns about vaccinations,* however, are much less understood and include:

- *They contain harmful heavy metals, chemicals, and weakened or dead viruses or bacteria.*
- *Injecting these substances into the body bypasses the immune system's defenses*
- *No studies have evaluated the long term safety of vaccinations.*
- *Serious questions exist about the effectiveness of vaccinations. There are no large subject studies that prove vaccinated children have less disease than unvaccinated ones. In Europe, where vaccinations are given much less, decreased illness rates were attributed to improved sanitation and nutrition.*
- *Many esteemed physicians and scientists believe that the short and long term dangers of vaccinations outweigh any possible benefits.*

Some believe that the vaccination program is a self-perpetuating source of business for the disease care industry. Those who work in hospitals often see children who need lifelong medical care because of serious vaccination side effects.

- *Vaccinations are a multibillion dollar industry; pharmaceutical companies exert powerful lobbying and educational influence on lawmakers, medical schools and doctors.*
- *Many serious illnesses and deaths have occurred in healthy children shortly after receiving vaccinations. Since 1990, over billions of dollars in damages have been paid to families whose healthy children died or developed strange maladies after getting vaccinations.*
- *Protocols now call for children to receive about 80 injections by school age. Surely even the staunchest defenders of vaccination programs must admit this is excessive.*
- *Immunity can be developed by other means, including breastfeeding, natural exposure, and natural health care.*

These concerns really hit home when you've seen just one child whose life has been seriously or irreversibly ruined after receiving vaccinations.

Renowned pediatrician Robert S. Mendelsohn MD, author of *How to Raise a Healthy Child In Spite of Your Doctor,* stated: "The greatest threat of childhood diseases lies in the dangerous and ineffectual efforts made to prevent them through mass immunization... There is no convincing scientific evidence that mass inoculations can be credited with eliminating any childhood disease... While the myriad short-term hazards of most immunizations are known (but rarely explained), no one knows the long-term consequences of injecting foreign proteins into the body of your child. Even more shocking is the fact that no one is making any structured effort to find out. Have we traded mumps and measles for cancer and leukemia?"

Children, the fastest growing population segment for the expanding pharmaceutical industry's products, are even supposed to get flu shots. The following are quotes from the manufacturers product insert for recent flu shots:

- *"There have been no controlled trials adequately demonstrating a decrease in influenza disease after vaccination with ___."*
- *"It is not known whether ___ is excreted in human milk. Safety and effectiveness of ___ in pediatric patients have not been established."*
- *"The virus is inactivated with ultraviolet light, followed by formaldehyde. Disrupted with sodium deoxycholate, 45 mcg. Hemagglutinin (HA). Each dose contains 25 mcg mercury." (Note: Formaldehyde is a known carcinogen while mercury is a known neurotoxin that has been linked to autism and other neurological conditions.)*
- *"___ has not been evaluated for carcinogenic or mutagenic potential, or for impairment of fertility."*

Regarding adverse events associated with influenza vaccines, the same flu drug literature stated: "Individuals were observed for three days after the flu shot was administered" in order to find out if there were adverse reactions." *What if a problem surfaces weeks or months later?* Further, "Because these (adverse) events are reported voluntarily from a population of uncertain size, it is not always possible to reliably estimate their incidence rate or to establish a causal relationship to the vaccine."

The list of adverse events reported include: "Lymphodenopathy, eye pain, photophobia, dysphagia, vomiting, influenza-like symptoms, rhinitis, cellulitis, muscle weakness, arthritis, tremor, syncope, Guillain-Barre syndrome, convulsions, seizures, cranial or facial nerve paralysis (Bell's palsy), encephalopathy, limb paralysis."

Flu vaccines for children? Who is watching out for our children's well being? If you thought it was the government and orthodox health care system, you're living in a dream world. People need to wake up to the reality of how much health care in the U.S. is controlled by profit-oriented businesses. We need to educate ourselves and protect our children. Who else will do it if not you and me?

Vaccines are the fast-food version of acquiring immunity, but much more dangerous. They are relatively cheap and quick, but can cause significant side effects and even death. Many people are uninformed about this topic or are too busy to take the safer route.

Our daughters were not vaccinated because we didn't feel the potential short and long-term risks were worth any possible benefits. We did everything we could to help develop their immune systems naturally: breast feeding, optimal diet, nutritional supplements, spinal and cranial bone checkups, common sense health habits, and sensibly avoiding people with acute illness.

Now in their 30s, neither contracted any significant childhood illnesses. Their lack of vaccinations caused no legal problems in school from kindergarten through college. Many states allow exemptions from vaccinations based on religious or philosophical grounds. I know numerous children of other doctors and patients who went the same route and were just fine.

Please take the time to educate yourself about this critical topic before exposing your children to so many potentially harmful injections. Here are a few quotes on the topic:

- *Ivan Illich PhD: "The combined death from scarlet fever, diphtheria, whooping cough, and measles among children up to fifteen shows that nearly 90% of the total decline in mortality between 1860 and 1965 had occurred before the introduction of antibiotics and widespread immunization."*
- *Philip Incao MD: "In my medical career I've treated vaccinated and unvaccinated children and the unvaccinated children are far healthier than the vaccinated ones... There is little or no objective research into the possible adverse effects of vaccines. There has never been a study comparing vaccinated to unvaccinated children. The only explanation for this is bias and political pressure."*
- *W.B. Clark MD: "Cancer was practically unknown until smallpox vaccination began... I have never seen a case of cancer in a non-vaccinated person."*
- *Tedd Koren DC: "Today the major threat to our children's health is not infectious disease but chronic illnesses of the immune, nervous, and other organ systems. We see epidemics of allergies, asthma, autism, developmental disorders, learning disabilities, attention*

deficit disorders and hyperactivity (ADD/ADHD), cancer, multiple sclerosis, cerebral palsy, eating disorders, diabetes, epilepsy, Tourette's syndrome, stuttering, anorexia and bulimia... the list is long and depressing. Most of these conditions were rare or unknown before mass vaccination and there is increasing evidence that it's not a coincidence that this is so."

- *Forbes Laurie MD: "I am convinced that the increase in cancer is due to vaccination."*

For more information, contact the National Vaccine Information Center at **nvic.org**. Recommended reading about vaccinations includes: *Childhood Vaccination: Questions All Parents Should Ask* by Tedd Koren DC; *A Shot in the Dark* by Harris L. Coulter PhD and Barbara Loe Fisher; *How to Raise a Healthy Child... In Spite of Your Doctor* by Robert S. Mendelsohn MD; *Vaccines: Are They Really Safe and Effective?* by Neil Z. Miller; *Vaccines* by Sherri Tenpenny DO; *The Sanctity of Human Blood* by Tim O'Shea DC.

The Bottom Line

The most important points in the *Natural Care* chapter include:

1. *Take time to educate yourself about natural ways to prevent and treat illness.*
2. *Recognize the risks associated with medication and surgery and only use these for emergencies*
3. *Develop a natural health care team to help you become and stay as healthy as possible*
4. *Use natural healing approaches, especially chiropractic, herbs, nutrition-based health care, acupuncture, integrative medicine, massage, and essential oil therapy.*

5. *Regularly check children and adults for spinal and cranial alignment, especially after physical trauma*
6. *Start babies off on the right foot with the 3 L's: Leboyer, La Leche and Lamaze*
7. *Educate yourself about the pros and cons of vaccinations. Learn about natural ways to strengthen the immune system of children and adults.*

Action Steps for Natural Health Care

List two action steps you commit to starting within 30 days:

1. ______________________________
2. ______________________________

List two action steps you commit to starting within 60 days:

1. ______________________________
2. ______________________________

List two action steps you commit to starting within 90 days:

1. ______________________________
2. ______________________________

R A D I A N T

Transcendence

Key #7
Transcendence

"If the doors of perception were cleansed, everything would appear to man as it is, infinite." —William Blake

Life on earth can *seem* so fragile and fleeting.

The word "seem" is a key one, however. As Blake's quote indicates, when you accurately perceive reality, you realize that life is infinite and magnificent. Even when it seems otherwise.

And that one realization can change your entire earth experience.

The seventh key is really very simple: you are an eternal being of energy/consciousness/spirit. Your real self cannot be hurt or destroyed.

The implications of this key are tremendously transforming, both personally and globally. You can handle all life's challenges and changes because you are an integral part of Life Source. You are in eternity *now,* not someday maybe.

Contrary to what you might have been told, you do not have to believe, say, or act any certain way to become one with the One. You already are – that's the life is set up. However, certain beliefs, words, and actions help you *remember* that your high nature and live as such.

Deeply knowing who you are can make your time on earth more heavenly *now and always* no matter what is going on around you.

All life events – even death and dying – make more sense from an enlightened perspective that glimpses more of the greater reality. Bodily death is just a gateway to another phase of forever. That's why other cultures use terms such as *changing worlds, dropping the body,* and *graduating.* These words remind us that we are forever beings living in a totally supportive and loving universe.

I know how difficult it is at times to grasp this great news. But it's possible and essential for radiant wellness.

Bill Pitstick, my dad and one of my best friends, passed on in 2017. He was always larger than life, happy, positive, and a great role model. Dad helped many people in many ways and was adored by his family. I felt very sad when he passed and still miss seeing, hugging, and talking with him.

However, my resolute knowledge of our eternal natures lightened my grieving. I was even able to *celebrate* his graduation into the next phase of life.

I continue to talk with him and listen for replies. I've had dreams and waking contacts with him that seem to be actual contacts. I know that only his outer shell fell away. Everything else – his love, huge heart, leadership, and rascal personality – continue on. I have no doubt that I will see him again more fully and look forward to that.

And, as I'll share later, he even handled dying like a champ.

What a gift to be able to go through life's toughest times with peace, acceptance and trust instead of excess upheaval, anger, and fear. That's one reason it's so important to really know your transcendent nature.

Synonyms for *transcendent* include extraordinary, absolute, whole, boundless, eternal, infinite, otherworldly, supernatural, and ultimate. These words describe the breadth and depth of our highest natures.

Before going any further, let me address an important topic. There are over 10,000 religions in the world and more than 38,000 denominations, cults and sects in Christianity alone. Conventional wisdom warns against discussing religion. Rest assured, this chapter is not about any particular religion but my best current understandings of life, death, and afterlife.

Death anxiety is a *pervasive fear* that keeps many people from living fully and joyfully now. Many people have serious concerns about death and afterlife, and they aren't satisfied with orthodox answers. I've been with many people as they or their loved ones were dying. They appreciated evidence-based information to augment their faith.

That's why I discuss transcendent topics. Documented clinical, scientific, and empirical evidence provides great comfort and support. Enjoying life and handling the tough times is easier when viewed from an informed and awakened perspective.

My book *Soul Proof* presents nine categories of evidence that you and everyone else really are indestructible beings of energy/consciousness.

1. ***After-Death Communications (ADCs):*** *Over 25 percent of people in general, 66 percent of widows, and 75 percent of parents whose children have passed on have experienced contact with their departed loved ones. Evidential and shared ADCs further indicate that they are more than wishful thinking or the imagination.*
2. ***Near-Death Experiences (NDEs):*** *This is the most publicized category of proof. Tens of thousands of validated cases strongly indicate that consciousness continues after physical death. Authenticated NDEs involving blind people and children are particularly impressive.*

3. ***Miraculous and Revelatory Encounters:*** *Angel contacts, miracles, and revelatory experiences further indicate that there is much more to life than the five senses can perceive. Miracles experienced by more than one person at one time have extra credibility.*

4. ***Scientific Input:*** *Double-blind, peer-reviewed, journal published, and statistically significant studies at major universities strongly suggest that communication with living souls can occur. In addition, many eminent scientists have strong beliefs about the reality of unseen dimensions.*

5. ***Peri-Natal Experiences:*** *Clinical and empirical evidence suggests that children can sense events before, during, and just after birth. Incoming souls have communicated with their biological and adoptive parents before conception. These verified perinatal experiences add more weight to the hypothesis that consciousness precedes birth.*

6. ***Evidential Mediums' Input:*** *A number of people with mediumistic abilities are considered authentic by physicians. Researchers at five different universities and centers have verified the ability of certain persons to reliably communicate specific information from those who have passed on.*

7. ***Cyclical Life Experiences:*** *Much evidence indicates that we live not just this one, but many different lives and includes: child prodigies, familiarity, xenoglossy, curative reports, similarities between lives, past life regression data, children's past life memories, and Dr. Ian Stevenson's research.*

8. ***First-hand Experience and Other Ways of Knowing:*** *This category includes: firsthand experiences; contributions from artists, writers and philosophers; intelligent design theory; and common sense. Input from this category further points to the data that we each are timeless beings of energy.*

Collectively, these categories provide impressive evidence that you are an eternal being having a temporary human experience.

———◆———

Many people have asked the following questions:

- *Who am I?*
- *Why am I here?*
- *What happens after I die?*
- *Is there a God?*
- *Why is there so much suffering?*
- *Once I know my spiritual nature,* ***how can I best live?***

My answers to these important questions come from contemporary evidence, my personal and professional experiences, and my best current understandings. I do not claim to have all the answers or the only answers, especially given the magnitude of these topics.

Who Am I?

The collective evidence clearly indicates that you are an ageless being of energy, an indestructible being of consciousness. That's from a dualistic view that sees separation among the various aspects of creation.

From a *non-dualistic perspective,* all life is interconnected and essentially one. From this viewpoint, you already are an integral part of and inextricably interconnected with Life Source. You are a vital part of life's never-ending but ever changing dance of energy.

In both viewpoints, you have a transcendent and enduring nature. It's a sweet deal.

Your timeless self is like your hand that is always present whether you are wearing gloves or not. You slip a glove (your body) on at birth and off at death, but your awareness is always there.

From our 21st century vantage point, we can evaluate the collective evidence and conclude that we are eternal beings of consciousness who are just visiting earth for a short while.

Why Am I Here?

It appears that souls choose this earth experience for five primary reasons: *loving, service to others, adventure, growth, and enjoyment.* This earthly journey may provide opportunities and experiences not possible in higher energy realms. The first letters of the words "service, adventure, growth, enjoyment" spell the word sage. This acronym is a reminder that we are visiting this physical plane for important reasons—for sage training. Let's examine the four.

Serving others is one reason we're here. Native American wisdom has long taught that all people have a "give-away," a special gift to impart at the right time.

Serving others benefits both the giver and the recipient. Ralph Waldo Emerson said, "It is one of the most beautiful compensations of this life that no man can sincerely try to help another without helping himself."

Some people feel *an inner emptiness* due to a lack of purpose or direction in life. A self-centered life devoid of service just doesn't feel right. The solution for this problem is simple: open your eyes and heart and see how life calls you into service.

Adventure is the next reason that we, as souls, come to such a challenging planet.

One morning years ago, I began rousing from sleep and was aware of a recurrent phrase in my mind. The phrase was: *this earth experience is a totally safe, meaningful, and magnificent adventure amidst eternity.* That's become one of my guiding themes.

Your time on earth can be seen as an exciting adventure when you remember your infinite nature. You can enjoy every aspect of life when *you really know* that life is ever-changing, but never-ending. You already know that everyone's story has a happy ending, even if it seems grim during the middle pages.

Many people enjoy books and movies with action and suspense. It's the same way in life. A constant sameness where nothing exciting happens would soon get boring so your soul signs up to experience adventures.

Every aspiring hero needs something to overcome such as a mean villain or great adversity. That's why fairy tales and legends of knights are such universally popular themes. Adventure allows you to expand your perceived limits and to find out just how powerful and capable you are.

Growth is the next reason that forever beings volunteer to visit a place like earth. *Advanced learning* is a huge motivation for visiting physical dimensions.

Just as you go through elementary, junior and senior high school, you likewise benefit from life's *gradational lessons.* Handling the challenges of this planet can powerfully assist consciousness raising. Difficulties help you work on your rough edges and discover what parts of yourself are not yet congruent with the Light.

As you have probably experienced, life's toughest challenges provide the biggest lessons. This physical plane is a *perfect classroom* for personal growth because of its density and struggles. It's like weight lifting: to develop bigger muscles, you lift more weight more times.

Challenging experiences provide perfect opportunities for developing spiritual muscles.

Enjoyment is the last reason why beings of consciousness visit this planet. Consider the myriad experiences available on earth that some take for granted: the feel of rain drops on your skin, the sound of waves on the water, views of sunsets and sunrises, fragrances of fresh flowers, tastes of fresh ripe fruit, the touch of a loved one's caress.

Life, whether on physical worlds or in non-earthly dimensions, is so full of exquisite richness and wonder. Why not enjoy the entire spectrum of creation?

As Joseph Campbell put it, "If you follow your bliss, you put yourself on a kind of track that has been there the whole while, waiting for you, and the life you ought to be living is the one you are living."

Loving, service, adventure, growth and enjoyment: that's a lot packed into one incarnation that lasts *only a blink of an eye* when compared to the span of eternity. That's why you're here.

———◆———

What Happens After I Die?

What happens after I die? That depends on which "I" you're talking about.

Your physical body will eventually cease functioning and turn to dust. Anyone who has spread the cremated remains of a departed loved one knows that. But your real self will continue on into the next phase of life without limitations of brain-based thoughts and perceptions.

The next question that naturally arises is: "What is the quality or nature of the afterlife?" Many of us were taught that there are only two possible outcomes after death: heaven or hell. But what does the collective evidence show?

The short answer is: what you experience after bodily death depends on your state of consciousness at the time of passing. That is, the quality of your afterlife experience will be determined by your beliefs, how you treated others, how balanced or imbalanced you were, your strong likes and dislikes, etc.

Much evidence points to *universal salvation,* an open-ended possibility for a harmonious afterlife for everyone. Input from near death experiences, evidential mediums, and firsthand experiences agree. These sources indicate that a magnificent state of being is always available now, after you die, and forevermore.

Is There a God?

The word "God" conjures up various meanings to different people so let's discuss that one a bit. There are various facets to God. When I was five years old, my parents showed me a beautiful sunset and I told them "It reminded me of God." That remark suggests a remembrance of a Source of beauty, love and power.

Near death experiencers have described this phenomenon as love, light, energy, wisdom and understanding this knows no bounds. They refer to this as the Light, the Source, and the Presence. Others have experienced this phenomenon via mystical experiences, out of body experiences, and life between lives sessions. All concur that *God is love.*

The God I'm talking about is the creative and sustaining force behind *the cosmos,* not just one isolated time and culture on earth.

And yet, at the same time, Creative Energy is *intimately connected* to each one of us. Lord Alfred Tennyson wrote, "Closer is He than breathing and nearer than hands and feet." Creator is like the sun and the various aspects of creation are like rays of sunshine. God is like the ocean and we each are like a drop of water.

For those seeking *scientific evidence* that a higher intelligence permeates all existence, read *The G.O.D. Experiments: How Science Is Discovering God In Everything, Including Us* by Gary E. Schwartz, Ph.D. He uses the acronym G.O.D. to indicate a Guiding, Organizing and Designing process that is operative at all levels of life.

My current favorite term – E.L.G.O.D. – builds upon Dr. Schwartz's acronym with the letters E and L that stand for Energizing and Loving. E.L.G.O.D. thus captures more of the attributes of this ultimately ineffable phenomena. The two additional letters, E and L, also honor ancient names for the Ground of All Being. El or Al – the root words of Elohim, Eloha, Allah, and other sacred names for God – meant The One or That One which expresses itself uniquely through all things.

This more complete image of the Divine answers many age-old questions. For example, it's common for people who are suffering to ask, "Why is God doing this to me?" or "Why did God take my loved one?"

Understanding that you are an integral part of Creator now and forevermore helps you remember that no separate sovereign power dictates what happens. However, we each – as eternal parts of the One – may choose to undergo certain experiences for the growth and service opportunities.

Please don't let anything stop you from *personally knowing* the living Source of all life. You can experience a peaceful and joyous relationship with *All That Is* via regular prayer, meditation, time in nature, spiritual study and trusting that still small voice within.

Why Is There So Much Suffering?

This question obviously needs to be asked. If there's a supremely present, powerful, loving, and knowing God – and we're each part of It – why is there so much suffering? Further, if we're all timeless beings of energy and a heavenly life is always available, why bother with this earthly experience that is so cruel and painful at times?

These questions primarily arise if you believe that there is any meaningful separation between you and God or anyone else. I don't now, but I used to.

Tony Robbins teaches that the quality of our lives is determined by the quality of the questions we ask. Instead of asking why there's so much suffering, perhaps a better question is: "How can I remain loving, peaceful, and clear during difficult times?"

The answer to that question may sound deceptively simple at first: cultivate an unshakable knowing that you are an eternal being in a totally supportive universe and live accordingly.

Might it be that souls purposely choose seemingly tragic, but *spiritually instructive lessons* by being paralyzed, molested, tortured, starved or killed? This viewpoint doesn't condone harming others or imply an uncaring attitude about such suffering. Certainly we all should do everything we can to alleviate human suffering. However, this perspective helps us understand that perhaps there are meaningful reasons for human woes.

In *Emmanuel's Book,* channeled by Pat Rodegast, Emmanuel says that suffering and strife are perfect backdrops for soul growth. He asks, "If this world were a perfect place, where would souls go to school? ... View your world as a transient place where souls choose to come because this is what they have selected as their mode of learning to the most minute detail... There is an overall plan of which you are not aware and to which you can only contribute by being who you are, doing your best, seeking your higher truth, and following your heart."

Buddha taught that one cause of suffering is *selfish desire.* When you must have something, you set yourself up for suffering. It's OK to *prefer* to be healthy and have a great life with material possessions, loving family and friends. But an enlightened person can live without them if need be and doesn't desperately have to have them.

Following the golden rule reduces suffering since inappropriate actions cause much imbalance on earth. In the movie *Oh God,* John Denver asked "God," "If you're so involved with us, how can you permit all the suffering that goes on in the world?" George Burns as God replied, "I don't permit the suffering—you do. Free will. All the choices are yours... you can love each other, cherish and nourish each other, or you can kill each other."

Here are some wise thoughts about suffering:

- *Bernie Siegel MD, says that afflictions heal and adversity opens you to a new reality. He calls these apparent setbacks "spiritual flat tires—unexpected events that can have positive or negative outcomes, depending on how we respond to them."*
- *Nietzsche: "That which does not kill me, makes me stronger."*
- *In* ***You'll See It When You Believe It,*** *Wayne Dyer, Ed.D., states: "I have a very strong belief that everything that comes into your life is supposed to, and every condition of your life is part of the perfection of it, and there's a blessing in all of it, and that there are no accidents, that it's a perfect—absolutely totally perfect—universe."*
- *Rabbi Harold Kushner, author of* ***When Bad Things Happen to Good People,*** *says God is on our side—even when it doesn't seem like it. Regarding terminal diseases and death by forces of nature, he stated, "Laws of nature don't make exceptions for nice people.*

Expecting God to spare good people from pain is like expecting a bull not to charge you because you're a vegetarian."

- *Elisabeth Kubler-Ross, M.D., wrote: "Life naturally begins when the soul, the entity, enters the physical body to start a new existence in the physical world. We are here to grow, to learn, to have all the experiences that the physical world can offer. And when we have passed all the tests, we are allowed to graduate and return back to our original home."*

Many other great teachers have addressed the question of suffering and given similar answers. This wisdom is reflected in an old African proverb: "The blessing lies close to the wound." There's a silver lining to every cloud when you look for it.

Thank God that we can grow and learn even during difficulties and tragedies. Remember your transcendent nature, live accordingly, and notice how the universe seems infinitely more hopeful, fair and safe even amidst suffering.

———◆———

Once I Know My Eternal Nature, How Can I Best Live?

How would you live if you knew *for a fact* that the real you – all the love, memories, energy, personality, uniqueness, and much more – doesn't die?

Five suggestions for enlightened living include:

1. *use spiritual practices*
2. *enjoy time with kindred spirits*
3. *engage fully in life armed with faith and knowledge*
4. *magnificently care for the temple of your soul*
5. *enjoy utopian living now—no matter what*

Regularly use spiritual practices to remember your timeless nature and enjoy life to the fullest. Utilize prayer, meditation, spiritual study and support groups. Benefit from worship, ritual, singing, chanting, time in nature, breath work, or practices like yoga.

A traditional salutation in India involves bowing, putting the hands together, and saying *namaste.* The bow recognizes meeting another high being who is another facet of the Creator. Bringing the hands together symbolizes seeing through the illusion of separateness and realizing that all life is interconnected.

The word means 'I honor the light within you; I recognize that place within each of us where we are truly one.' This wonderful spiritual practice takes only a few seconds and reminds both people about how life is set up.

In Thailand, a word for 'hello' is *sawadee* which also means "I see Buddha." In China, the word qi or chi means "breath, life force, spirit." In Japan, the word is *ki;* in India *prana.* These words recognize the God within each person. The language of these cultures have built-in reminders about our true essence.

Native Americans viewed life as a daily walk with Great Spirit.

Their youth undertook a vision quest, spending several days alone in nature while searching for guidance. As challenges arose, elders asked them, "How does this relate to your vision?" When someone died, they called it *changing worlds.*

The Bible points to the day when all people will understand their infinite natures and realize, "O death, where is thy sting? O grave, where is thy victory?" It teaches us to "gird our loins" with truth so we can fight a good fight and run a fast race while on earth. These metaphors speak to the importance of spiritually preparing ourselves for life's inevitable challenges.

Enjoying time with kindred spirits is another way to be fully in this world but remember there is much more to life.

Bertha had been a patient of mine for many years. As she grew quite old, I knew it was just a matter of time before she or a loved one passed on. We sometimes talked about the evidence that life does not end at death. I wanted to ensure that she was ready for life's biggest change and could face it without fear.

At one early morning appointment, Bertha didn't look well. Her eyes were red, she looked tired and her posture was drooped. "What's wrong, Bertha?" I asked.

"Oh, my husband died," she said.

"I'm so sorry. When did that happen?" "About four hours ago," she replied.

"Four hours? Bertha, we appreciate you keeping your appointment. But under these circumstances, we would understand why you couldn't make it."

"I know," she said, "That's what my family said, but I told them that I couldn't think of anyone I would rather be around at a time like this than you."

What a compliment and what a great lesson about how to handle grief. When you or your loved ones are dying, surround yourself with those who can *see through the illusion of death* – even a little bit. Lean on those who know, without a doubt, that you will see your departed loved ones again.

Better yet, don't wait until someone is dying. Regularly enjoy time with others with open hearts and minds. This will help you develop a rock solid soul group so you are prepared for whatever arises.

Engage fully in life armed with faith and knowledge so your life can be like an airplane trip. Knowing who you are allows you to enjoy the flight of this life, to relax and enjoy each special moment despite occasional turbulences. And when your soul transitions to its next destination, you can be assured of joyful reunions with loved ones you might not have seen for awhile.

In the past, people had to rely upon faith alone. Faith is good, but faith supplanted by convincing evidence is even better. From this 21st century perspective, we have an unprecedented knowledge base with which to accompany our faith.

Magnificently caring for the temple of your soul is what this book is all about. We've discussed how the quality of your time on earth is directly affected by how well you treat yourself. You can be a bright light in this world, not just a flickering candle flame, but an awesome torch that brightens everyone's day. Optimally caring for yourself helps you do that on all levels, always and in all ways.

Enjoy utopian living now to demonstrate the greatest benefit of knowing your transcendent nature. You can be a shining example of how an enlightened human can look, feel, and be.

When asked what we can do about all the problems facing humanity, Buckminster Fuller answered, "Live with as much integrity as you can". Having integrity means being honest, giving it your best shot, and doing the right thing. Can you imagine how great life will become as more people live with integrity? Let it begin with you.

After you die, you'll experience a life review, a replay of your key moments – both favorable and regrettable – while on this planet. The life review is designed *to teach and help you* – not punish, shame or criticize. Will your life review be a work of art or an embarrassment? It's up to you and it's *not too late* to record a masterpiece.

When you change worlds, you will be reunited with departed loved ones and other soulmates. Will you be proud of your track record while on earth? Your kindred spirits will give you a 'high five' or a 'Dutch rub' depending on how you lived. It's all in a spirit of love and growth, but wouldn't it be better to have a celebration?

Use images such as proudly reviewing your life and getting high fives to help you *soar* through life's puzzling predicaments and challenging changes. Live an illuminating life that deeply touches and inspires others.

You can enjoy utopian living this moment and forevermore. You can always experience heaven on earth, even during difficult times and even while dying. Sound impractical? I've witnessed many amazing demonstrations of this, including my dad's dying.

Dad didn't have an easy life at times. In his later years, he had lung, bladder, skin, and blood cancer. He also had open heart surgery twice. Despite all this, he never complained and was very happy and positive. Later, dad turned his suffering into an asset while volunteering at hospitals. He could comfort patients better than anyone because he had been through so much, but was still going strong.

At age 80, dad was diagnosed with severe leukemia and given two to four months to live with a prognosis of shortness of breath, bleeding, and extreme fatigue. But he said, "Don't feel bad about this. Everyone has to die sometime. The Lord and I have an agreement. I'm going to move on when it gets too bad."

He always handled life's challenges head on and decided the only way to win this one was to check out as soon as possible. Dad had a prior near-death experience after his second open-heart surgery and was given an opportunity to enter the Light. He declined because he wanted to finish some service projects and spend more time with my mom and his family.

So we figured he already had the ticket to the next realm in his hand; he only had to hand it to the conductor. He crossed over *just eight days* after his diagnosis, an awesome display of how much control we have in life and death.

During his last waking hour before passing on, it was obvious that his life force was slipping away and he was feeling the bliss of living in *fuller awareness* of the greater reality. The hospice nurse said that he wasn't on any medication that would cause euphoria or delirium.

Here's how Dad described how it felt: "I feel the best I ever have in my entire life. Everything is very smooth as if I'm covered with plastic. Everything feels soft. It's soft all around me and I feel soft—like a new towel that hasn't been washed yet."

Other excerpts from among his last words:

- *"If something in life doesn't work out how or when you think it should, don't worry about it. Everything happens in God's time and way."*
- *"Don't be afraid of dying or anything in life. The Lord will never put more on you than you can carry."*
- *"I've had such a great life, so many wonderful experiences, a loving family and so many great friends. I'm so blessed."*

We talked, laughed and cried until he felt tired and wanted to take a nap. "You guys are talking me to death," he said.

Vintage Bill Pitstick humor.

We all gave him a big hug and kiss. He told us to watch for a hawk on the drive home. Dad loved hawks and always spotted them wherever he went. He said, "I love you all," gave us a big wink, and closed his eyes for the last time. What an exit!

On the drive home, a huge hawk flew so close in front of us that we almost hit it.

Here are four of the many important lessons I learned from my Dad:

1. *Love with all your heart and don't hold back.*
2. *Let your inner light shine brightly and serve others with every fiber of your being.*

3. *Enjoy every precious moment of every day, even the little things and the rainy days.*
4. *Always remember that there's nothing to be afraid of since you are always walking with God/Universe/Spirit.*

That's right, my friends, you're not alone while attending this earth school. You have incredible inner potentials, helpmates and friends. You have a Higher Energy Assistance team that is always there to love, comfort, assist and guide you. And, always and without limit, is the Light. For all this, there is hope—no matter what is going on in your life. Even dying.

As Kenneth Caraway said, "There is no box made by God nor us but that the sides cannot be flattened out and the top blown off to make a dance floor on which to celebrate life."

Since dad's physical death, several members of our family have experienced inexplicable events: fragrances, doors opening and shutting, objects being moved. Mom was pinched on the behind when no one else was in the house. On several occasions while talking to him, she felt the mattress push down as if someone were sitting beside her. These signs comfort and energize us. They remind us that life continues on seamlessly, no matter what outward changes occur.

God is throwing a marvelous party, but most people are afraid to show up, let alone dance. With resolute knowledge that you are a forever being, your life can increasingly become an impressive demonstration of how amazing a human incarnation can be.

———◆———

The Bottom Line

The most important points in the *Transcendence chapter* include:

1. *Make it a priority to deeply know your true nature and live accordingly*
2. *Be empowered by the fact that you are a wise, infinite, special and powerful being.*
3. *Remember that you are here for important reasons.*
4. *Be assured that life continues on after death.*
5. *Develop a firsthand relationship with your Higher Power.*
6. *Be comforted by the evidence that even accidents and tragedies are important and purposeful parts of life.*
7. *Regularly enjoy meditation, prayer, study, time in nature and kindred spirits to remind yourself about the greater reality.*
8. *Use the **Radiant Wellness** keys to optimally care for the temple of your soul and enjoy a wondrous life now and always.*

Action Steps for Transcendence in Your Life

List two action steps you commit to starting within 30 days:

1. ____
2. ____

List two action steps you commit to starting within 60 days:

1. ____
2. ____

List two action steps you commit to starting within 90 days:

1. ____
2. ____

Afterword

An old Buddhist proverb states: "To know and not do is really not to know." Now you know.

Start taking action steps today to unleash your fullest potentials. Become a health nut, a self-actualizing person, and a spiritually awakened human. Devote a few hours each week to educate yourself and practice healthy lifestyle habits. Doing so will pay enormous dividends.

Your life can be outstanding in every way. It's not luck or just good genetics. It's a *conscious decision* to become all you can be no matter what it takes. Consistently follow the keys over time and watch your life radically improve. Do it for yourself and do it for others. *The world is waiting* for you to share your greatest gifts.

Nature teaches important lessons if we pay attention. My neighbor planted bamboo eight years ago and I watched those shoots turn into a small bamboo forest. Roots from his bamboo plants eventually grew into my yard and sent up shoots each spring, but I mowed over them.

After a few years, I decided to let the shoots grow in a confined area. Within just a few months, many 30-foot high bamboo plants had shot up. It was an amazing demonstration of how deeply entrenched roots can support rapid and tremendous growth. Humans are the same way. Regularly using these keys creates a firm foundation that can launch the life of your dreams.

Another bamboo lesson occurred last winter when we had a severe ice storm. Weighed down by the ice accumulation, two of the huge bamboo plants actually broke. So much for the saying that bamboo bends, but doesn't break.

Humans are like that as well. Even though we have a miraculous body and brain, we have a breaking point, a physical limit of unlikely return. Don't let yourself get to that point, please. Start now before you reach a point that is impossible or very difficult to come back from.

You can increasingly realize and demonstrate how wise, special and powerful you are. You can make your life a work of art and let your inner light shine brightly. Radiant. That's how you're supposed to be and how you can be.

In addition to improving yourself, please share this information with others. You now understand powerful principles and strategies for positively transforming body, mind and spirit. Don't keep them a secret!

May you fully enjoy life and powerfully bless others!

Introduction to Appendices

I've assembled self care and natural care recommendations for the most common health problems. Again, a disclaimer...

Note: This information is not designed to replace medical care and does not claim to diagnose or treat any disease. These strategies may assist your body to regain more normal functioning and heal itself. My recommendations are not supported by large medical studies, especially those funded by the pharmaceutical or disease care industry.

Whole food nutritional supplements are listed for each set of symptoms. Suggestions for supplements are based on my experience of helping many thousands of people during the last thirty-three years in holistic private practice.

The whole food and herbal supplements are from Standard Process / MediHerb and can not currently be shipped outside the 50 U.S. states and Puerto Rico. If you live elsewhere, you can visit StandardProcess.com to learn more about the quality and combination of nutrients and hopefully find them in your country.

As discussed in the Natural Care chapter, I strongly recommend that you have a team of health care practitioners for children, and if symptoms for an adult are severe and chronic. However, the programs I've outlined may help symptoms with moderate severity and shorter duration.

The numbers after each product – for example, Catalyn 6 – denote the dosage per day. Unless noted otherwise, supplements are best taken with two or three meals. Calcium products are best taken at dinner and bedtime to increase utilization. Supplement doses are for average size adults; adjust accordingly for a much larger or smaller adult. Children should take to of the dosage.

Because they come from concentrated whole foods, these products are extremely safe. However, holistic programs often lower high blood pressure, high cholesterol, high blood sugar, abnormal hormone levels, clotting times, and other important factors. Your medical doctors should know that you are starting a holistic program so they can decrease your medications as your body regains normal functioning and wellness.

Many people are eventually able to stop taking medications altogether, even after many years of taking drugs. However, you should not do that without medical supervision.

All of the products listed in the appendices are available for purchase at my office:

Dr. Mark Pitstick
Radiant Wellness & Chiropractic Center
234 N. Plaza Blvd. Chillicothe, OH 45601

To order, write to that address or email us at:
center@radiant101.com

The easiest way to order Standard Process and MediHerb products is through their Patient Direct program. Contact my office to get the code to allow this transaction.

My office staff can not take orders or answer any questions by phone since they are busy assisting the doctors.

Products that can be ordered from my office include:

- ***Standard Process*** *whole food supplements*
- ***MediHerb*** *supplements*
- ***21 Day Purification Program***
- ***Chlorella, Cilantro,*** *and* ***Homeopathics*** *to detox chemicals and heavy metals*
- ***Protein powders*** *from* ***Standard Process*** *and* ***Garden of Life***
- ***Green powders*** *from the same two companies*
- ***Joyful Body,*** *an essential oil combination for pain, inflammation, and spasm*
- ***Sinus Relief, Super Neti,*** *and* ***Respiratory Relief*** *– colloidal silver containing products for sinus and lung conditions*
- *Nebulizer for delivering a fine mist of* ***Respiratory Relief*** *into the lungs*

Some products, for example, the massage unit from *Homedics* and sinus rinse kit from *Neil-Med,* can be purchased at most pharmacies. We do not sell those.

There are two stages of supplementation:

1. ***Therapeutic:*** *you need to take more products at a higher dosage until imbalanced, weak, and stressed organs regain normal functioning*
2. ***Wellness:*** *after you are much healthier, you need fewer products and lower doses to stay well*

Even if they are not listed in a particular appendix, three wellness supplements are always highly recommended since they provide necessary nutrients for the entire body: *Catalyn 6, Cod Liver Oil 3, Trace Minerals B12 (3)*`

Note: except for severe and chronic cases that require more supervision, I work with a limited number of people to oversee their holistic healing program. This can be done in person, by phone, or with Zoom. If you want this service for yourself or a loved one, contact me at ***center@radiant101.com***.

Appendix A: ADD / ADHD

A twelve-year old boy was recently brought to our office for holistic health care. Chris suffered with symptoms that included behavioral outbursts, poor grades, and difficulty focusing. Joe, a thirty-two year old, also wanted help with his impulsivity, irritability, and forgetfulness. Despite the difference in their ages, they had two things in common: they were both diagnosed as having ADD (Attention Deficit Disorder) and were given two prescription drugs.

Their medical doctors hadn't asked about exercise, diet, stress levels, supplements, or sleep habits. They just prescribed two drugs. Is that 21st century health care?

Medications used to treat this syndrome can be dangerous and don't address the cause of the problem. Common side effects include nervousness, trouble sleeping, loss of appetite, weight loss, dizziness, nausea, vomiting, or headache. Symptoms of psychosis, heart attack, stroke and even death have been linked with these drugs.

ADD / ADHD is a syndrome—a group of symptoms that consistently occur together—not a disease. Those symptoms are the body's way of communicating that one or more factors are out of balance. When the imbalances are addressed, the symptoms go away. The causes of this syndrome can include:

1. *The mother was deficient in nutrients or had food allergies during pregnancy*
2. *Premature birth, being a twin, or born oversized*
3. *Neck trauma such as being born with the umbilical cord around the neck*
4. *Food allergies, most commonly to dairy, wheat, sugar, and corn*
5. *Genetics since 80% of ADD cases are boys*
6. *Wasn't breastfed but was given artificial formulas*
7. *Antibiotics given that created abnormal flora balance in intestines*
8. *Low blood sugar due to too many carbs and not enough protein and good fats*

9. *Vaccinations, especially when baby has side-effects soon after the shots*
10. *Poor self-image due to put downs by frustrated parents and teachers*
11. *Diet of processed, poor quality, and chemical-sprayed food or junk food. Excess sugar, especially artificial sweeteners, are another cause.*
12. *Excess stimulation from video games, TV, etc.*

In years past, coalminers took a canary in a cage with them. When the canary became sick, they knew the air quality was poor and it was time to get out of the mine. Similarly, youngsters who develop symptoms such as those associated with ADD are often sensitive. Their brains are trying to communicate that something is wrong, thus the symptoms.

In the U.S., the topsoil used to be at least three feet deep and contained all of the minerals that are needed. Now it's usually only six inches deep and even that is depleted of key nutrients so our food can't contain them. Throw in a bunch of pharmaceutical drugs—a pill for every ill—and excess chemicals and heavy metals and the stage is set for brain-related symptoms to occur often.

Your child might be quite bright but can't show it due to ADD symptoms. It's been said that Thomas Edison, Albert Einstein, and Winston Churchill all would have been diagnosed with this syndrome had they lived in this era.

The solutions for this syndrome involve addressing the causes above:

- *Avoid dairy, wheat, corn, and sugar for 90 days*
- *Eat 3 healthy meals per day with sufficient protein and limit carbs/sugar*
- *Avoid processed junk food, especially those with food coloring and chemicals*
- *Minimize over-stimulating TV and video games*

- *Chiropractic adjustments if needed to remove pressure from spinal cord*
- *Exercise and activities to channel extra energy*
- *Get a nutritional assessment to determine if excess chemicals and heavy metals are affecting the brain and / or hormonal system and how to best minimize them.*
- *Most importantly, reverse specific nutritional deficiencies by taking the following whole food supplements from Standard Process:* ***Cod Liver Oil (3 per day), Cataplex B (6), Catalyn (6), Trace Minerals B12 (3), Organically Bound Minerals (3), Tuna Omega Oil (3),***

If you or a loved one has ADD / ADHD symptoms, there is hope. Improvements are usually noticeable after just a few weeks. Nearly all cases respond very well when parents oversee the healing program for just ninety days. Adults also usually respond quite well—but not as quickly as children—when they follow the healing program consistently over time. After improvement, dietary restrictions can usually be relaxed and fewer supplements are needed.

By the way, with the help of his parents, Chris followed our program and began improving within weeks. Several months later, he is off his prescription drugs and is getting better grades. His teachers can't believe he's the same boy because he's doing so well. Joe was on the program for 3 months before noticing significant improvement, but he's very happy with his results. That's 21st century health care, addressing the roots of the problem versus giving dangerous drugs.

Appendix B: Bone Strength

In the U.S., about 45% of post-menopausal women have decreased bone density. The rate for men is increasing, especially for those taking prescription drugs for GERD. Bone density tests are described with a T-score for three groups:

- **T-score from 0 to -1.0**: *low normal bone density (slight concern warranted)*
- **T-score from -1.0 to -2.5**: *osteopenia (increased risk for bone fractures)*
- **T-score below -2.5**: *osteoporosis (should be very concerned)*

Medications given for GERD can cause spontaneous fractures in men as young as fifty years old. *Proton pump inhibitors* given for indigestion prevent the release of stomach acid, thereby decreasing normal breakdown of minerals and increasing incidence of hip fractures. Lower stomach acid levels may also allow harmful bacteria to enter the intestines and cause colitis.

Drugs given for osteopenia and osteoporosis can interfere with bone remodeling and may increase density but not strength. Over time, this interference with normal bone physiology can lead to bone death and spontaneous fractures in middle-age adults.

Recommended natural healing methods to increase bone strength include:

- ***No Smoking:*** *Smoking draws calcium from the bones*
- ***Limit Alcohol:*** *no more than one or two servings per day*
- ***Avoid Drugs:*** *certain medications deplete the body of calcium, especially when taken for many years. These include steroids, thyroid drugs, antacids, and GERD medications.*
- ***Exercise:*** *weight-bearing exercise is needed to increase bone density. Walking, aerobic machines, and resistance training (with yoga, bands or weights) stimulate new bone formation. Do for 30-45 minutes, 4-5 times per week.*

- ***Diet:*** *More vegetables, raw nuts and seeds that contain calcium and other minerals: sesame seeds, kelp, agar, almonds, carrots, spinach, okra, tomatoes, garlic, parsnips, applies, broccoli, eggs, beans, string beans, citrus fruits and potatoes, salmon, molasses, and certified raw or organic milk, yogurt and cheeses. Avoid soda pop and excessive red meat. Minimize coffee, fatty foods, white sugar, white flour.*
- ***Therapeutic supplements: f****or 3 months, take Calcifood 6, Cod Liver Oil 6, Zypan 3 – 6, Cal-Ma Plus 3. Then, for one year: Calcifood 4, Cod Liver Oil 3, Zypan 3. Cal-Ma Plus 1 per day with 1 week on, 1 week off.*

Appendix C: Cholesterol

Eminent medical doctors such Julian Whitaker M.D., Mark Hyman M.D., Al Sears M.D., and Joseph Mercola, D.O. agree with holistic physicians like me and Bruce West D.C. The *cholesterol scare is a scam* propagated by Big Pharma that controls much of the medical research. The disease care industry also profits obscenely when people unnecessarily use drugs to lower cholesterol levels.

Read articles by these doctors to understand that cholesterol-lowering drugs are dangerous and are rarely needed. (Rare cases with a genetic defect called familial hypercholesterolemia are an exception.) Contrary to what you may have been led to believe, there is no proven correlation between cholesterol levels and heart disease and mortality rates. That is, people who have heart attacks are just as likely to low, normal, or higher cholesterol levels.

This is a very serious topic for you and your loved ones. Statin drugs (Lipitor, Zocor, Crestor, Vytorin and others) have been shown to *increase the risk* of heart failure, diabetes, cancer and liver damage. *Side-effects* of these drugs include fatigue, muscle weakness, muscle pain, decreased memory, suicidal behavior, sexual dysfunction, digestive problems, neuropathy, depression and more.

Healthy lifestyle habits for those who want to control their total cholesterol, HDL, LDL and triglyceride levels safely and effectively include:

- ***21 Day Standard Process Purification Program:*** *this can significantly lower high levels in just 21 days*
- ***Don't smoke;*** *minimize alcohol if you use at all*
- ***Exercise at least four times per week*** *with interval training methods*
- ***Follow the Real Food Way of Eating***
- ***Avoid foods*** *containing white sugar and white flour; read labels*
- ***Minimize grains*** *and fruits and use only those from healthy sources*

- ***Eat plenty of eggs and meat*** *from organic, grass-fed sources and wild caught fish. Also regularly eat raw nuts and seeds (hemp, sesame, chia, sunflower) & avocados*
- ***Use healthy oils:*** *olive, coconut, and fish*
- ***Avoid unhealthy oils:*** *trans-fat and vegetable oils, especially reused*
- ***Reduce stress*** *by relaxing, enjoying leisure time, and a good night's sleep*
- ***Take whole food supplements*** *as listed below for optimal body functioning*

***In general, recommended supplements include*:**

- *A-F Betafood (6), Linum B6 (6), Cholaplex (6), Black Current Seed Oil (4) for high total cholesterol level*
- *Super-EFF (4), Immuplex (6), Cataplex B (6), Magnesium Lactate (3) for low HDL levels*
- *Linum B6 (3), Diaplex (9), Cataplex B (9) for high LDL levels*
- *Linum B6 or TOO (6), Diaplex (9), Cataplex B (9) for hi triglycerides and pancreas support*
- *Cataplex F (6), Thytrophin PMG (4) for hi triglycerides and thyroid support*
- *Cholacol 3, Cholaplex (9), Cholacol II (9) for hi triglycerides and liver support*

As always, you should consult with your health care team, especially if following the above program doesn't help normalize your lab values in 90 days.

Appendix D: Diabetes

Natural healing methods can often help type II diabetes (DM II). Many people have controlled this health problem via healthy diet, improved lifestyle habits, and wholefood supplements that help the pancreas and liver function more normally. DM I cases are more difficult to normalize but, in most cases, blood sugar levels become more stable and overall health improves.

In most cases after several months of natural care, DM II patients are able to *wean off their prescription drugs* with their medical doctor's supervision.

Jack's blood sugar was chronically around 400 despite being on three medications for diabetes. An evaluation of his diet showed that he ate too many carbohydrates and sugar. We taught him the healing diet and recommended four whole food supplements. Within two months, his blood sugar was normalizing to the low 100's in the morning. After four months, he was able to get off all of his medications and, several years later, has no problem at all. Six years later, his blood sugar is normal without any medications.

This is what is often possible when the root problems are addressed.

Orthodox medical approaches consider there to be no cure for DM II. Their drug treatment is designed to control the symptoms, not get to the cause of the imbalance. However, drugs for DM II have a long list of potential side effects: muscle pain or weakness; numb or cold feeling in your arms and legs; trouble breathing; feeling dizzy, light-headed, tired, or very weak; stomach pain, nausea with vomiting; or slow or uneven heart rate. There are many more possible side-effects that can ultimately be fatal.

That's why it's wise to *address the underlying causes of the problem* versus taking potentially dangerous drugs that only manage, not cure.

Natural healing methods for DM II include:

1. *Get chiropractic adjustments for normal nerve supply from the brain to the pancreas, liver, and other organs*

2. *Mildly exercise – for example, walking – 30 minutes five days a week*
3. *Lose weight if necessary (see Appendix ___)*
4. *Use the Real Food Way of Eating (see Diet chapter). You may need to follow the Healing Phase for six months and may need to limit your fruit to low glycemic varieties even during the Maintenance Phase.*
5. *Especially eliminate sugar, pop, and high fructose containing products*
6. *Take whole food supplements: (take one of each before each meal and at bedtime):* ***Diaplex 4; Cataplex GTF 4; Cataplex B 4; Pancreatrophin PMG 4***
7. *Also take the three maintenance supplements: Catalyn 6, Cod Liver Oil 3, and Trace Minerals B12 (3)*
8. *Monitor your blood sugar more closely since the above program often sharply lowers glucose levels. Keep a record of your levels and show your medical doctors so they can lower your medications accordingly.*

For additional information, read these articles by Julian Whitaker M.D. and Joseph Mercola D.O.

http://www.drwhitaker.com/4-natural-type-2-diabetes-treatments/

http://www.mercola.com/diabetes.aspx

Appendix E: Flu Prevention and Treatment

The days are shorter and the sun is lower in the sky. As a result, you receive less sunlight necessary for vitamin D production that is so important for a strong immune system. Throw in a few sugary holidays, weather changes and strange viruses from those receiving flu shots and the stage is set for getting the flu.

Are flu shots the answer? You can decide for yourself based on a recent flu vaccine manufacturer's *product information.* To summarize:

1. *No proof exists that flu shots decrease the frequency or severity of the flu*
2. *The vaccines contain harmful products such as mercury and formaldehyde*
3. *Serious potential side-effects such as convulsions, paralysis and much more can occur after getting the shot*

What can you do about it *naturally*? Plenty! Here are 3 natural ways to boost your immunity naturally, inexpensively and safely...

- *Practice optimal self-care as outlined in Radiant Wellness*
- *Eat only minimal sugar especially during stressful times and weather changes*
- *Use wellness supplements: Catalyn 6, Cod Liver Oil 3, Trace Minerals B12*
- *Get extra vitamin D during winter months in cold climates: Cataplex D 3 and a total of six Cod Liver Oil per day.*
- *Obtain extra sunlight during winter months by sitting by a window on a sunny day with your skin exposed. Also walk outside to get some sun exposure. Using blue light therapy is also helpful.*
- *Practice commonsense precautions when around someone with the flu*
- *Get a nutrition-based healing evaluation to ensure that your body and various organ systems are strong, balanced*

If you do start to experience flu symptoms, start the *Immune Enhancement Program* (Appendix H) as soon as possible. This approach has helped many people recover after *just one day* of a flu instead of suffering for a week or more. Many of our long-term chiropractic and nutrition patients notice that everyone else in their office or family gets sick, but they don't. So you aren't a helpless victim. You do have control over your health.

Appendix F: GERD / Chronic Indigestion

Natural healing methods can often help common symptoms. Chronic indigestion is also referred to as acid reflux, heartburn, acid indigestion and gastro-esophageal reflux disease (GERD). In this condition, partially digested food and liquid from the stomach backs up into the esophagus. This can cause great discomfort and eventually damage the stomach / esophageal tissue with an increased risk of cancer.

Backing up of stomach contents can be due to: overeating, overweight, excess stress, too much alcohol, inadequate chewing, too many spicy foods, excess sugar, smoking, overuse of antacids, carbonated beverages, estrogen replacement therapy (ERT), and hydrochloric acid deficiency. Some prescription drugs lower the gastric juice acidity and prevents the stomach from properly digesting food. Check Drugs.com to see if any of your medications have this side effect.

Other underlying causes include lying down or bending over soon after eating, fatty and fried foods, swallowing too much air when chewing, poor food combinations, aspirin and NSAID (prescription or OTC anti-inflammatory) usage, gall bladder problems or removal, nutritional deficiencies, tight-fitting clothing, pregnancy, and food allergies / intolerances.

Rarely, a true hiatal hernia exists in which the upper stomach protrudes through the diaphragm. This may respond to visceral adjustments and exercises to strengthen the diaphragm muscle. Severe and chronic cases may require surgery.

Symptoms can range from mild and occasional to severe and frequent. They may include: regurgitation, angina-like pain, difficulty swallowing, belching, gas, bloating, shortness of breath, sore throat, nausea, chronic cough, and a sense of fullness.

Standard medical treatment includes antacids, acid neutralizers, and acid suppressors such as Rolaids, Tums, Zantac, Prilosec, Prevacid and Nexium. All of these weaken the stomach acid and, while perhaps providing temporary relief, often worsen the underlying condition.

Natural healing methods include:

1. *Chiropractic spinal adjustments for normal nerve supply from brain to stomach. Visceral adjustments can ensure normal position of the stomach.*
2. *Addressing the above causes*
3. *Nutritional supplements: Gastrex (3 – 6) and Okra Pepsin E3 (3 – 6) taken 30 minutes before each meal; Zypan 3 - 6, Multizyme 3 – 6, Pituitrophin PMG 3*

Appendix G: Heart Health

Frank, a 62-year-old chiropractic patient, came to our office for several years and did some of the right things for his health. He ate a fairly healthy diet and managed his stress after retiring from a very demanding job. A serious athlete when younger, he exercised three times per week and also sweated a lot when working outside. However, there were three factors that ***weren't healthy*** for his heart.

1. ***He took*** *a cholesterol-lowering drug that his medical doctor prescribed even though his levels weren't high. (Many integrative medical doctors consider a total of less than 260 to be normal.) One of the known side-effects can include cardiomyopathy or weakening of the heart muscle. Another is muscle pain and spasm. This was Frank's number one symptom; I showed him the side-effects of that drug in Drugs.com but he fully trusted his medical doctor.*
2. ***He took*** *medication that his medical doctor prescribed for high blood pressure even though it wasn't elevated. After age 60—unless there is diabetes or kidney disease—a blood pressure below 150/90 is considered normal by many medical doctors. His was 130 / 90 before the drugs were prescribed. So he was taking a second drug that he didn't need but that had more potential side effects.*
3. ***He didn't take*** *whole food supplements to feed his heart with key nutrients that are needed for the heart to work well over time. The heart is a muscular pump that beats over 115,000 times per day. It uses minerals and other nutrients to function properly, but can't work right if those are deficient.*

I talked to Frank many times about getting evaluated with Nutrition Response Testing (NRT) and see if his heart muscle had the necessary nutrients to function normally. He always replied that his medical doctor said his heart was "just fine." Besides his occasional back pain that was relieved by spinal adjustments, his only symptoms were muscle spasms in his calves and upper back after exertion.

Did you ever get a "Charlie horse" or muscle cramp in your calf or foot and feel like you would die? Well, when you get a muscle spasm of your heart muscle, you can die. That's what happened to Frank. He was feeling fine, but keeled over with a heart attack and died. I guess his medical doctor was wrong about his heart being "just fine."

And no wonder. The average medical student receives less than 4 hours of nutritional training. We have spent many hundreds of hours attending post-graduate seminars and studying the subject. Medical doctors provide wonderful care for emergencies such as broken bones, ruptured appendices, and twisted bowels. But for many common problems, including heart disease, their "treatment" is useless at best and deadly at worst.

Some medical doctors are waking up to this fact. David Katz, MD, director of the Yale University Prevention Research Center, says there is no drug, and there never will be any drug, that can reduce the burden of chronic heart disease. How effective is medical treatment? For people over 65 years of age who were in the hospital for heart failure, 67% were readmitted and 36% died within one year. For those with a heart attack, those numbers are 50% and 25%. I don't like those odds and neither should you... but you need to take responsibility to prevent and, if necessary, naturally treat heart disease.

Fortunately, just six factors are needed to prevent most heart problems:

1. *whole food diet and pure water as described in our Healing Diet handout*
2. *moderate exercise such as brisk walking and light exercise 3 times a week*
3. *quit chewing or smoking tobacco*
4. *regularly relax and use breathing exercises to avoid excess stress*
5. *proper nerve supply from the brain to the heart itself via chiropractic adjustments*

6. *heart-healthy, whole-food nutritional supplements when neededBruce West, DC, and his team of integrative health care providers have helped over 30,000 heart patients return to health using natural methods, especially nutrition. He cites a January 2015 Medscape article citing heart doctors who are coming out of the closet and admitting that, in most cases, drugs, heart surgeries, stents, angioplasty and other dangerous and costly procedures don't work. To learn more, visit HealthAlert.com*

Does your heart muscle need extra nutrients? You might if you sweat a lot or have in the past. It's also more likely if you are or have been on blood pressure or GERD drugs, or others that cause mineral loss. Finally, anyone after age 40 should take extra 'cardio-tonic' nutrients because the heart has pumped nearly two billions times. I recommend getting a personalized nutritional evaluation if you have any heart problems. See below for a great preventive heart nutritional program.

I can't bring Frank back. I wish I had gotten through to him and he was still alive. I'm sure his wife, children, and grandchildren feel the same way. But, hopefully, others will learn from his untimely death so they can enjoy more quality and quantity of life. And that will impart more meaning to his life and death.

Preventive and Wellness Nutritional Supplements for the Heart
General: Cardio-Plus 6; Cataplex B 3; Min-Tran 4; Cod Liver Oil 3, Calcium Lactate 6 - 10; Cyruta Plus 3 - 6

Other: Magnesium Lactate 2 - 4 (if muscle cramps); Hawthorne 2 – 3 and HerbaVital 2 - 3 (if fatigue); Cataplex E2 3 - 6 (if chest pain)

Appendix H: Immunity Enhancement Program

The following natural treatments—*at the first sign of a scratchy throat, runny nose, cough or sneeze*—can greatly reduce the severity and length of the symptoms.

1. ***Extra rest:*** *sleep in, go to bed early, and cancel nonessential activities.*
2. ***Talk to yourself:*** *tell your body that you hear its message and you will get more balanced so it doesn't have to go through a full cleansing crisis.*
3. ***Pure water and food:*** *drink 1/2 of your body weight in ounces of water per day. No junk food, sugar, wheat, fried or processed foods, or dairy products.*
4. ***Sinus rinse*** *eliminates excess mucous, kills microorganisms, and aids clearer breathing. The salt water that does not burn or sting. Use 2 - 4 times daily*
5. ***Thymus thump technique*** *stimulates blood cells that fight infection. Firmly tap over the upper sternum for one minute, four times per day.*
6. ***Avoid antibiotics*** *and other drugs as much as possible to allow normal functioning of the body, and prevent super-resistant microorganisms.*
7. ***Natural remedies :***

   a. ***Congaplex,*** *two every hour until improved; then 6/day for 1 week (1/4 to ½ of all doses for children)*

   b. ***Immuplex:*** *1 per hour until improved, then 3/day for 1 week*

   c. ***Cod Liver Oil:*** *6/day until improved, then 3/day for 1 week*

   d. ***Sinus Relief spray*** *(if sinus involvement; contains colloidal silver) every hour until improved, then 4 times per day for 1 week*

e. ***Respiratory Relief*** *(if lung involvement; contains colloidal silver): 3-5 cc in nebulizer 4 times per day until cough improves, then 2/day for 1 week.*

8. ***Immu-Tea:*** *drink 2 to 3 servings of per day. Mix 2 cups of filtered water, 2 minced garlic cloves, and 2-inch length of grated ginger root. Bring to boil and cover for 5 minutes over low heat. Sprinkle cayenne pepper as tolerated, about ¼ teaspoon. Add juice of 1 lemon and 1 TB. honey.*

Discuss these natural strategies with your health care providers while you and your loved ones are healthy so you are prepared when an illness begins.

Appendix I: Joint Disorders

Common joint problems can often be prevented and helped with safe, affordable, natural and effective approaches:

1. ***Weight Loss:*** since extra weight stresses the hip and knee joints, use the *21 Day Purification Program* and the *Real Food Way of Eating.*
2. ***Drink Water:*** ½ of your body weight in ounces per day of pure filtered water
3. ***Joyful Body*** (or *Glory Be, CBD* for more severe and chronic pain) are essential oil combinations formulated by Andy Lee, RN, LAc, CCA. For topical use only; rub firmly onto painful joints 2 – 4 times per day. *These plant oils help relieve pain, spasm and inflammation. For topical use only. Shake and firmly rub one spray* onto painful joint *2 – 4 times per day.*
4. ***Traction:*** *Lay on your back and relax completely. Have someone gently traction your knee and / or hip joints by grabbing above the ankle and pulling. Then, shake the leg up and down several times, then back and forth while tractioning. For the shoulders, traction by grabbing on the elbow side of the wrist joint. Do once per day.*
5. ***Ice:*** *place a damp washcloth over joint(s). Place a large bag of ice and cover with a folded towel. Leave on for 20 minutes. Repeat 2 - 6 per day depending on severity of pain.*
6. ***Muscle/Trigger Point Massage:*** *(see Appendix ___)*
7. ***Resistance Training:*** *for the involved area; ask an assistant at your local gym for guidance. A stationary bike is excellent for the hips and knees. Use low tension; start with 5 minutes and build up to 20", three times per week*
8. ***Ergonomics:*** *for example, observe good waking posture; use padding when kneeling on a hard surface; alternate sleep positions on both sides and your back*
9. ***Whole Food Supplements:*** *Glucosamine Synergy 3, Calcifood 3, Cod Liver Oil 3, Zypan 3, Calcium Lactate 6,*
10. ***Stretching:*** *(see Activity chapter)*

Note: in addition to the home care methods outlined above, you should receive chiropractic adjustments or physical therapy to ensure normal joint alignment and range of motion. You may also need one or more therapies such as laser therapy, taping, bracing, and ultrasound.

Appendix J: 'Mental' Symptoms

I am no stranger to these so-called 'mental' symptoms. One of my first childhood memories is trying to help my mom because she cried and was depressed so much. Other family members suffer with these symptoms and take medications with side-effects such as tremors and impaired mental function for them. Others have used excess alcohol, nicotine, coffee, and sugar to self-medicate and feel better temporarily.

I have a moderate predisposition to depression and have worked hard—especially during times of great stress—to stay balanced and happy. As a youth, I felt depressed and antisocial at family gatherings until I connected my massive sugar intake with the mood changes. When my first love broke up with me at age 21, it felt as though I were falling into a deep, dark hole with no hope of escape. I briefly thought about running my car into a bridge embankment to escape the pain but, fortunately, didn't act on that impulse.

Over the years, I've developed powerful self-care strategies that serve me well. These natural methods can also help you and your loved regain your health and life.

There's a silver lining to every cloud. Seeing my family members suffer motivated me to search for sensible solutions to these common symptoms. As both a clinical psychologist and a holistically oriented chiropractic physician, I've worked with many patients who suffered with these. In my experience, *almost all cases* of 'mental' symptoms can be successfully treated with Safe, Affordable, Natural and Effective (SANE) methods IF patients follow a holistic program over time.

The Problem

Incidence of depression in the U.S. is approximately 10% with a 5% worldwide rate. Approximately 3000 people commit suicide each day because of depression. News reports regularly tell about a celebrity, athlete or famous person who "has it all" but still suffers with 'mental' symptoms. According to Julian Whitaker M.D., of the school shooters whose medical records have been made available, all suffered with depression and other mental symptoms and were on psychiatric drugs. The financial and personal costs are beyond measure.

Eighteen-year-old John suffered with severe depression, anxiety and insomnia for several months. He had several plans to kill himself if his symptoms didn't improve soon. Luckily, his family saw his struggles and sought health care guidance. Their medical doctor recommended an anti-depressant drug and sleeping pills. I recommended a nutrition-based method to detect what stressors and deficiencies were causing his symptoms. Fortunately, his family chose door #2.

John had been exposed to lots of chemicals as a child. He also had a chronically poor diet and mineral deficiency after losing eighty pounds in a short period of time. Both factors were affecting his brain function and his symptoms were red flags to communicate that something was wrong. I gave him whole food nutritional supplements to help remove the chemicals and provide key nutrients needed for normal brain function. He felt 50% within a few days, 75% better in a week and 95% better in two months. He resumed work, school and a normal life without taking potentially harmful drugs for the rest of his life.

I've been shocked to see how many young people suffer from 'mental' symptoms. It's an epidemic that needs to be addressed by caring health care professionals who aren't inordinately influenced by the disease care industry that requires high profits to please shareholders.

'Mental' symptoms affect all age groups.

While in theology school, I worked at a suicide prevention and counseling center. The toughest cases were elderly women who were severely depressed, anxious, and suicidal after decades of an empty or abusive relationship. They had no resources, no hope, and were in too deep of a hole to recover. I'm sure that some of them did kill themselves or died from cancer or some disease in which the body attacks itself.

Years ago, I worked with Bonnie, a middle-aged woman who was very depressed and anxious. Her father died a year before and she had dealt with the grief. However, her church taught that those who didn't believe a certain way would suffer in hell forever. Her father hadn't been "saved" before he died and, she believed, would fry for eternity. Bonnie blamed herself for not getting through to him and felt partially responsible for what she thought would be his endless fiery torment.

The Causes

In my experience, the most common causes of depression, anxiety, panic attacks, and obsessive-compulsive disorder symptoms are:

1. *Nutritional deficiencies, especially after: one or more pregnancies, excess sugar and alcohol intake, severe stress, and a chronically poor diet. People of non-Caucasian ancestry seem to be especially vulnerable to the ravages of poor diet. I believe this is because – until very recently – those races enjoyed active lifestyles, adequate sunshine, and a real food diet.*

   Fifty years ago, most doctors didn't understand that pregnancy creates nutritional deficiencies and, sadly, the situation hasn't changed much since then. Most mothers are told to continue taking their pre-natal vitamins, as though those few synthetic nutrients will do the job.

   Post-pregnancy nutritional deficiencies can cause depression shortly after birth or a few to many years later. While giving their history, many middle-aged women have told me, "My symptoms started shortly after my second child was born and I've never been the same since." They often have a potpourri of chronic symptoms that few doctors can solve. So they are given "happy pills" or have their reproductive organs cut out, but—in the long run—that just worsens the situation.

2. *Food allergies and offending foods: GMO, chemical-laced non-organic foods, processed junk food. Wheat, sugar, soy, corn, and dairy products from factory-raised cows are usually the worst offenders.*
3. *Overgrowth/imbalance of microorganisms in the body (viruses, bacteria, yeast or parasites)*
4. *Excess electromagnetic fields (EMF) from 'dirty electricity' sources*
5. *Excess chemicals due to the 2000 chemicals we're exposed to daily*
6. *Toxic or heavy metals from body care products, home cleaners, and many other sources*
7. *Skin trauma*—scars from surgery, cuts, animal bites, body piercings, tattoos or IV sites—that interfere with normal sympathetic nerve transmissions
8. *Excess waste products and toxins in the body, especially eliminative organs—the liver, colon, skin, lymphatic system, lungs and kidneys*
9. *Chronic insomnia and fatigue*
10. *Misaligned spinal and cranial bones that put slight pressure on the spinal cord and brain.*
11. *Boredom/creative discontent due to not following ones purpose/ missions.*
12. *Side-effects of prescription. Antidepressant drugs, for example, can have major side-effects including increased suicidal or homicidal behavior. That's why the FDA requires a 'black box warning' on anti-depressant drugs. Psychiatry, the least scientifically based branch of medicine, still uses primitive, hazardous therapies such as electro-convulsive shock therapy to treat depression so beware.*
13. *Prolonged and excessive stress that imbalances the adrenal glands, brain and immune system.*
14. *Chronically poor relationships that are unfulfilling, negative or abusive.*
15. *Negative influences from fear-based religious denominations*
16. *Lack of exercise and all the negative results of being out of shape*

17. *General poor health due to poor self-care such as smoking, excess alcohol, drugs, inadequate rest, too much time on the computer/ video games/TV, etc.*
18. *Medical emergencies: tumors, severe diseases, and other conditions can cause 'mental' symptoms and may require orthodox medical care. Medical treatment is miraculous and indicated when emergency or crisis conditions are involved. However, for many common symptoms, the disease care approach can cause worse problems and doesn't address the underlying causes.*
19. *Emotional Crises: symptoms can occur after the death of a loved one, loss of job, disability, financial loss, chronic stress, empty nest syndrome, etc.—especially if a person is not balanced. These create short or long term stress, but natural healing approaches can usually help.*
20. *Lack of Sunshine: in cold northern climes during the winter, lack of sunshine can lead to lower vitamin D levels and less activity outdoors. In areas predominated by cloudy and gloomy skies, that may also contribute to more depression.*

Keep in mind that a person can be affected by more than one cause at the same time. That's why holistic health care considers all the underlying causes and treats the whole person. It also explains why many health-care specialists—who primarily focus on one bodily system—often don't understand the core causes and resort to treating the symptoms with drugs.

When seeing these different potential causes, some people feel overwhelmed at the prospect of making so many changes. That's why you need a coach, a health care professional who can evaluate which ones are affecting you. You don't need to change everything but you do need to address the major causes.

Here are a few *real-life cases* of patients who regained their health and their lives again when the root causes were addressed...

Larry experienced depression, anxiety, brain fog and severe headaches for many years. His history revealed several falls and auto accidents in which he had hit his head. I found significant misalignment of the upper neck vertebrae and skull bones. These were exerting slight, but impactful pressure on his spinal cord and brain. After a few weeks of specific and gentle adjustments, Larry started feeling better. After a few months, his symptoms were gone.

Kathy had been a chiropractic patient for many years and had just given birth to her second child. I could tell something wasn't right as soon as she walked into my treatment room. "I just wanted to say good-bye," she said. "I'm going to drive my car in some direction until I run out of gas and then I'll start walking through fields and woods until I die." Fortunately, I knew how to help. She didn't need a spinal adjustment that day; she needed *replacement of vital nutrients* that had been lost during her second pregnancy. With a *personalized program* of whole-food supplements, she quickly regained her normal cheery disposition. Years later, we shake our heads at how close she came to making a poor decision from an imbalanced state of mind.

June had several causes that combined to cause symptoms of depression and anxiety. She smoked too much and her diet was poor. Her marriage wasn't bad, but it wasn't meeting her needs. She was bored and had too much time on her hands. We tuned her up with nutrition-based healing and chiropractic care. She quit smoking and began exercising. With her renewed energy, she started working part-time and spent more time with family and friends. She communicated her needs for a better relationship with her husband and, to her surprise, he responded positively. After addressing these causes, her 'mental illness'... well, I guess it just flew out the window, because she doesn't have those symptoms anymore.

Holistic Solutions

1. *Nutrition-based healing methods as discussed in Natural Care chapter. They can usually address the # 1 – 8 causes listed above. Suggested supplements are at the end of this appendix.*
2. *Spinal and cranial adjustments (Natural Care chapter)*
3. *Release stuck emotions. (Awareness chapter)*
4. *Have happy, loving relationships. (Awareness chapter)*
5. *Exercise (Activity chapter)*

6. *Identify and follow your heart-felt missions (Awareness chapter)*
7. *Get into the swing of life. Excess isolation can cause depression and anxiety so – even if you don't feel like it – interact with others at community events, church, a safe neighborhood bar, yoga and meditation center, etc.*
8. *Enjoy the Real Food Way of Eating. (Diet chapter)*
9. *Avoid chemicals and heavy metals as much as possible. (Inner Cleanse chapter)*
10. *Counseling from a licensed therapist and / or minister (Awareness chapter)*
11. *Have an integrative medical doctor* on your health team. (*Natural Care* chapter)
12. *Be your self. (Awareness chapter)*
13. *Centering practices (Awareness chapter)*
14. *Adequate sunshine: See Appendix M: Seasonal Affective Disorder*
15. *Visualize what you want. (Awareness chapter)*
16. *Use Ying Yang Balance, an essential oil combination to assist calming and clarity created by Andy Lee, RN, LAc, CCA. For topical use only. Lightly rub a 2 x 2 inch area onto each forearm 1 – 2 times per day.*
17. *Develop a personal relationship with Creator. (Transcendence chapter)*

Summary

Again, remember that there can be *multiple causes of 'mental' symptoms* so work with your health care team to identify all of the causes and design your healing program accordingly.

And, again, please don't feel overwhelmed by all the causes and solutions. Enlist the help of supportive family and friends. Choose one cause and address it to increase your energy and clarity. Then use that boost as *a springboard* to tackle another cause. Your body and mind will thank you for just small improvements and reward you with more peace, joy and vitality.

You can do it. The world needs your fullest gifts and you deserve to feel happy, healthy and energetic.

Suggested Nutritional Supplements

Catalyn 6, Cod Liver Oil 3, Trace Minerals B12 (3), Cataplex B 3, Cataplex G 3, Mintran 6 (or more as needed for anxiety and insomnia), *Tuna Omega Oil 3*

Consult a nutrition-based practitioner if this general program and other recommendations haven't helped within 90 days.

Appendix K: Muscle Spasm

Many people suffer with chronic muscle spasm and tension. Over time, these can form *trigger points* that become hard, knotty, and very painful. They can range in side from a pea to a ping pong ball and are most commonly found on the hips, shoulders, and upper traps. Also known as *myofascial bundles,* this fibrotic scar-like tissue can cause radiation of pain into the head, arms, and legs. They can cause muscles to go into spasm after minor activities such as twisting or bending.

Trigger points mimic other conditions and often are not properly diagnosed or treated. The good news? With appropriate treatment and diligent self-care over time, this condition usually significantly or completely improves.

Causes of trigger points include: past physical trauma (auto accidents, falls, sports or work injuries, etc.); excess stress; chronic misalignment of spinal and skeletal bones; poor waking and sleep postures such as sleeping too much on the same side of your body; abnormal ergonomics, that is, bodily stresses due to improper lifting, desk height, computer monitor positioning, etc.

Home treatment should initially be done *daily* for severe cases, every other day for moderate ones. After your pain improves, continue treating the areas three times per week for two months *to completely resolve the trigger points* so they don't become chronic or intermittent. Use the following home treatment methods:

1. ***Ice for 20 minutes:*** *twice per day with six times per day if severe pain.*
2. ***Massage unit:*** *we use the Homedics© brand available at most pharmacies for about $45. The contact points vibrate 30,000 times per minute to reset and relax chronic areas of spasm. Alternate light to firm pressure directly over the trigger points in several different directions. The patient should relax and breathe through this treatment since it can hurt a lot. Use daily for two weeks, then three times per week for two months to fully heal the area.*

3. ***Joyful Body*** *(or Glory Be, CBD for more severe and chronic pain) are essential oil combinations formulated by Andy Lee, RN, LAc, CCA. These plant oils help relieve pain, spasm and inflammation. For topical use only. Shake and firmly rub one spray onto involved muscles 2 – 4 times per day.*
4. ***Stretching:*** *twice per day in a pain free range (see Renewal chapter)*
5. ***Nutrition:*** *Calcium Lactate 8, Cod Liver Oil 3, Magnesium Lactate 2*

Note: In addition to your homework program, you need *corrective chiropractic adjustments* to ensure normal alignment and range of motion of your skeletal and spinal bones. Severe cases of muscle spasm may also require muscle stimulation, low level laser-light treatment, or deep massage therapy.

Appendix L: Post-Pregnancy Nutritional Deficiencies

Karla was a thirty-eight year old mother who had recently given birth to her second child. She had been a chiropractic patient for many years so, when she came into the office, I could tell that something wasn't right with her. When I inquired, she broke down crying and admitted that she had been extremely depressed, nervous and exhausted. She couldn't focus mentally, didn't sleep well and was planning to kill herself. Her medical doctor recommended anti-depressants, but those made her feel worse due to several side effects.

I explained to Karla that *symptoms caused by post-pregnancy nutritional deficiencies* were common, especially for mothers after one or more pregnancies—whether they went full term or not. The developing baby pulls many nutrients from the mother's body. Breastfeeding, although highly recommended, takes additional nutrients from the mother. Finally, recovering from caesarean section surgery is additional stress to the body. If the lost nutrients are not replaced, and they seldom are, the mother's physical and mental health can go downhill from there.

After childbirth, women may be advised to continue taking a pre-natal vitamin, but those are *synthetic* (made from chemicals, not whole foods), *fractionated* (contain just a few vitamins and minerals instead of the broad spectrum of nutrients as found in nature), *high dose* (instead of lower doses found in real food) and *poorly absorbed* (not usable or even recognizable by the body.) Most supplements bought in stores or pharmacies are like this.

Fortunately, we caught Karla's problem before she made a poor decision from her (nutritionally) imbalanced state of mind. Within a few weeks of taking a personalized program of whole food supplements, she was back to her normal self. She now enjoys her family, her job, and life in general—just like she used to.

While working with many thousands of patients during the last 40 years in hospitals, mental health centers and holistic private practice,

I've interviewed many women who reported that their health spiraled steadily downward after one or more pregnancies. *"Ever since my second baby," they say, "I've never been the same."*

These symptoms are due, in part, to chronic post-pregnancy nutritional deficiencies. Mothers may not have experienced post-partum depression, but they still had a lack of key nutrients. Over time, their symptoms piled up—depression, anxiety, fatigue, weight gain, insomnia, brain fog, poor hair and nails—and their physicians didn't know where to start. So they were prescribed medications from each specialist who doesn't see the big picture.

Please share this information with ***mothers of all ages*** since some older women become physical and emotional wrecks due to decades of nutritional deficiencies. The perimenopausal stage (before, during and after menopause) can become a nightmare if there are preexisting nutritional deficiencies *and* hormonal imbalances.

Menopause can be much smoother than most women experience. As the ovaries shut down their hormone production, the adrenal glands and the rest of the endocrine ideally pick up the slack. However, many women have weak or imbalanced pituitary, thyroid and/or adrenals. So when menopause arrives, it can be like a roller-coaster from hell instead of an occasional bump in the road.

I've helped many women reverse symptoms of night sweats, hot flashes, mood swings, insomnia, fatigue, overweight, poor nails and hair, and weak bones. These are the most common symptoms that occur during this age range but it doesn't have to be this way. Tuning up the hormonal system and providing optimal nutrients gives these women their lives back and makes the husbands happy too.

By the way, the more pregnancies—including miscarriages—a woman has, the more likely she is to suffer afterward with physical and "mental" ailments. These symptoms may occur soon after the pregnancy ends or may take years to show up.

Medical doctors who don't understand the impact of post-pregnancy nutritional imbalances may think these women are "head cases" and prescribe an anti-depressant. The side-effects of these mind-numbing drugs include fatigue, weight gain and a long list of others including increased homicidal and suicidal behavior. The ensuing downhill slide affects everyone: the mother, the children, the husband, and the marital relationship. Very common but, fortunately, easily treated.

The 4 ways to know if you might suffer with these nutritional deficiencies include:

1. *You have been pregnant one or more times*
2. *You suffered depression, anxiety, or other symptoms shortly after delivery*
3. *After delivery, especially two or more times, you slowly went downhill with a growing list of physical and "mental" symptoms*
4. *You are having significant symptoms as you approach or go through menopause or around time of your menstrual cycle*

Holistic Solutions

1. *Fine-tune your body with the approaches discussed in Radiant Wellness*
2. *Get a nutrition-based healing evaluation if your symptoms are chronic or severe*
3. *For less severe cases, use the following supplements for 90 days: Catalyn 6, Cod Liver Oil 3, Trace Minerals B12 (3), Calcium Lactate 6, ForTil B12 (3), Symplex F6*

Appendix M: Seasonal Affective Disorder

Winters in northern areas can cause a number of symptoms due to vitamin D deficiency. The term *seasonal affective disorder* (SAD) describes a combination of *mood swings* (depression and fatigue) and *sleep disorders* (not sleeping well or sleeping too much.) Other symptoms linked with too little vitamin D include frequent colds / flus, joint pain, and muscle cramps. If you suffer with any of these symptoms, you may benefit from the natural remedies below.

1. ***More sunshine:*** *your body produces vitamin D when it gets sunshine. During winter months, you can expose your skin to sunlight three ways:*
   - *a. Sit in front of a window while wearing a bathing suit so lots of skin is showing that can soak up the rays*
   - *b. Take a walk or other outdoor exercise with as much skin exposed as possible; roll up your sleeves and let the sun shine on your face*
   - *c. Go south, even for just a long weekend, to a warm sunny area. You'll feel better looking forward to the trip, during, and afterwards.*
2. ***More vitamin D:*** *most vitamin D supplements contain only one type (D3) of a processed form that is of little use to the body. I recommend two products to give your body dozens of forms of D from naturally processed food sources: Cod Liver Oil 3 – 6 and Cataplex D 2 – 4.*
3. ***Fake sunshine:*** *I recommend the Apollo or Phillips brand of GoLite blue light therapy. They cost about $120, but mine has lasted ten years so far. I shine it on me while I'm working on my computer. I do not recommend tanning beds based on warnings from dermatologists and personal experience with skin cancer exactly where my skin touched the tanning bed.*
4. ***Anticipation:*** *remember that it will get warmer and sunnier again someday. Look forward to those days and, when they arrive, really enjoy them.*

5. ***Whole body tune-up:*** *cold, rainy/icy, and gloomy weather create thermal stress on your body. If any organ or system—your hormonal system, for example—isn't strong, the weather might be the last straw that triggers a serious imbalance. Symptoms are your body's way of telling you that something is wrong. Chiropractic, acupuncture, and nutrition-based care can help.*
6. ***Wellness nutritional products:*** *in addition to the Cod Liver Oil and Cataplex D, take Catalyn 6, and Trace Minerals B12 (3)*

Appendix N: Sexual Functioning

Sexual dysfunction symptoms are quite common after age 40 but it doesn't have to be that way. For men, symptoms can include reduced or lack of: sexual desire, achieving an erection, maintaining an erection, and orgasm. For women, the list includes reduced or lack of: interest, lubrication, enjoyment, and orgasm.

It's difficult to address all the factors involved in this short appendix, but here are my basic recommendations:

1. *Realize there is nothing to be embarrassed about. Communicate with your spouse or partner about any problems in your relationship, get counseling if necessary, and change for the better.*
2. *Get sufficient rest and relaxation on the day of lovemaking. Sexual arousal works best when you're relaxed, rested, and happy.*
3. *Be more creative during foreplay: a glass of wine, a backrub with oil, different positions, sharing fantasies, etc. Pornography is not a good idea for many reasons as discussed in article #30 at* SoulProof.com
4. *Look, smell, and be attractive and energetic as possible with exercise, diet, and other strategies discussed in Radiant Wellness. Decreased sexual interest and functioning can occur if one or both partners let themselves go downhill physically.*
5. *Check* Drugs.com *to find whether any of your prescription drugs could cause decreased sexual interest or performance. Tell your medical doctor that you want to be on no medications or, if absolutely necessary, as few as possible.*
6. *Get a medical check-up to make sure there are no severe health problems that are contributing to your lack of optimal sexual performance.*
7. *Use natural healing methods –unless there is a true medical crisis – such as chiropractic, acupuncture, and nutrition to improve cardiac, prostate, hormonal, and other systems. These can improve sexual functioning, general vitality, and relieve pain that can diminish a healthy sex life.*

8. *Tune up your body and brain with a nutritional healing program. Your body will focus on survival—not sexual enjoyment – if one or more of your organs (heart, brain, hormonal) are weak, stressed, and imbalanced.*
9. *Whole food supplements: Symplex F 6 (for women) or Symplex M 6 (for men), Tribulus 2, Fortil B12 (3), Catalyn 6, Cod Liver Oil 3.*

As always, seek more supervised care if the above program doesn't significantly help within 90 days.

Appendix O: Sinus Symptoms

Safe, affordable and natural remedies can often help sinus congestion, drainage, pressure, headaches, and recurrent infections. Recommendations include:

1. *Avoid smoking and other sinus irritants—second hand cigarette smoke, fumes, dust, heavy pollen, grass particles, and chemical sprays—as much as possible:*
2. *Minimize or avoid junk food, dairy products and sweets.*
3. *Drink a lot of water: your body weight in pounds divided by 2 in ounces per day*
4. *Optimize eliminative routes as explained in Inner Cleanse chapter so your sinuses aren't overloaded with waste removal.*
5. *Sinus massage technique for sinus headaches while lying on your back. Briskly massage the sinuses above and below the eyes. Next, apply firm pressure and tap with your fingertips over these areas, especially the most tender spots.*
6. *A saltwater nasal rinse technique helps kill microorganisms and mobilize secretions. I recommend the Neil-Med brand. For the frontal sinuses above the eyes, tilt your head back during the rinse. Use once or twice per day until your symptoms improve, then wean down to once per week maintenance. Use at the first sign of a sinus infection or after exposure to irritants under #1.*
7. *Detoxify to remove excess toxins from your sinuses, liver, kidneys, bowels, and lymphatic system. The Standard Process 21 Day Cleanse assists removal of chemicals, heavy metals and excess wastes.*
8. *Receive corrective chiropractic care for optimal nerve supply to the sinuses and TMJ function. Massage relaxes muscles to aid lymphatic drainage of head and neck.*
9. *For chronic sinus symptoms, obtain a nutrition-based healing evaluation (see Natural Care chapter) to address the underlying causes.*

10. *Whole food supplements that often help include:*

    a. Allerplex: 4 - 6 per day

    b. Antronex: 6 - 9 per day

    c. Sinus Relief: one spray up each nostril every 30 or 60 minutes if you have yellow or green mucous when you blow your nose; decrease frequency, then halt use as sinus infection improves.

    d. Congestion Relief: 1 spray each nostril as needed for congestion; decrease frequency, then halt use as sinus infection improves.

    e. SuperNeti liquid undiluted, one dropper each nostril while supine 2 – 4 times per day; decrease frequency, then halt use as sinus infection improves.

Appendix P: Smoking Cessation

You can enjoy a healthy and vibrant life free from addiction to tobacco. The following program has helped many people overcome this destructive habit.

1. *Do you really want to quit? If not, visit people in nursing homes who suffer with emphysema. Also consider that people exposed to second hand smoke are much more likely to develop lung problems. So stopping helps you and your loved ones.*
2. *Know that nicotine is as addictive as heroin. That's why it's not easy to break the habit. The first week after quitting is usually the toughest so be prepared.*
3. *Set a date to quit; birthdays or special dates add additional power. Get extra rest, eat well, and be good to yourself during this time of withdrawal.*
4. *Tell friends, family and co-workers you are quitting and ask for their help.*
5. *Drink 8 or more glasses of water per day to flush your system of toxins.*
6. *Remove all cigarettes, matches, and ashtrays from your home.*
7. *If family member(s) smoke, keep their packs wrapped in a piece of paper. If the urge to smoke becomes too great, you must first write down the date, time, why you want a cigarette, and why you want to quit smoking. Going through these steps will usually delay the impulse to smoke and help you resist the urge.*
8. *Have action steps ready when the urge to smoke grows: take walks, call a nonsmoker friend, pray, chew gum, relax, take deep breaths or scream into a pillow.*
9. *Stopping all at once is best. If that seems too difficult, wean down by 3 cigarettes per day every two weeks, then quit completely when you're only smoking 3 per day.*
10. *If past attempts to become a nonsmoker haven't been successful, consider acupuncture or hypnosis to assist you.*

11. *Take the following supplements to help successfully quitting: Mintran 6 – 20 per day to help anxiety, Catalyn 6, Cod Liver Oil 3, ForTil B12 (3), Tuna Omega Oil 3, Cataplex B (4)*
12. *Be reassured that most people who successfully break the tobacco habit do so after several "failures." If you start smoking again, don't feel guilty or berate yourself. Set a new date and try again until you succeed.*

Appendix Q: Thyroid Balance

Balancing thyroid function is very important and requires skillful supervision. Please consult a nutrition-based healing practitioner (see *Natural Care* chapter) if you suspect thyroid imbalance.

Hypothyroid symptoms may include dry skin, brittle nails, thinning hair, depression, fatigue, weakness, being too cold, pear-shaped body with weight and fat gained in buttocks and hips. *Hyperthyroid* symptoms may include: insomnia, weight loss, weakness, fatigue, rapid heart rate, feeling too hot, and nervousness.

Avoid Thyroid Poisons & Aggravating Factors:

- ***Chlorine and Fluorine:*** *use whole house water filtration system*
- ***Pesticides:*** *avoid exposure to household pesticide sprays*
- ***Estrogen:*** *is highly thyroid inhibiting; whenever possible avoid hormone replacement drugs and estrogenic herbs such as black cohosh, licorice, soy, pennyroyal, and sage.*
- ***High Dose Synthetic Vitamins:*** *for example, beta carotene inhibit thyroid function*
- ***Radiation and Mercury;*** *from x-rays, CT scans, dental amalgam fillings*
- ***PABA:*** *a synthetic B vitamin, also present in sun tan lotions*
- ***Thyroid hormones*** *that can shrink the thyroid, suppress the pituitary, induce osteoporosis, and increase cancer rates*
- ***Unsaturated Oils:*** *avoid liquid oils except olive and flax oils*
- ***Soy Products:*** *soybeans, tofu, soy protein, soy milk, tempeh, etc.*
- ***Vegetarian Diets:*** *protein deficiency inhibits thyroid function*
- ***Liver Damaging Substances:*** *alcohol, prescription drugs, cigarettes, processed foods, poor quality water.*

***General Supplements**: Symplex F (M for males)* 3 per day; *Organically Bound Minerals* 3; *Calcium Lactate* 6; *Cod Liver Oil* 3; *Thytrophin PMG* 3; *Thyroid Complex* 2

***For hypothyroid**: Prolamine Iodine 2;* **avoid** raw cruciferous vegetables – especially juiced (broccoli, cauliflower, cabbage)

***For hyperthyroid**: Mintran* 6 or more until symptoms improve; 8 oz. cabbage juice daily

Appendix R: Tremors and Neuro-Muscular Disorders

Three months ago, Ralph started treatment at our office for severe tremors of his hands and feet. His medical diagnosis was Parkinson's Disease, but Ralph wanted a second, natural health care-based opinion.

He noticed that when he bent his head backwards, his shaking ceased. He had suffered two severe neck injuries, as a child and ten years ago. As a result, the normal curve in his neck—that houses the spinal cord as it leaves the brain—was curved the wrong way. So for fifty years, he's had pressure or distortion on his spinal cord. Over time, that disrupted the normal nerve connection between his brain and muscles.

In addition, his muscular and nervous systems are very deficient in key nutrients needed for properly functioning. After just three months of Nutrition Response Testing and specific chiropractic care, his shaking is nearly gone and he feels much better.

Over the years, we've helped a number of patients with these neuromuscular disorders—Multiple Sclerosis (MS), Parkinson's, Lou Gehrig's Disease, Multiple System Atrophy (MSA), and essential tremors. These cases were diagnosed by neurologists at highly respected medical centers such as Mayo Clinic.

(I should emphasize that our success rate is good if patients come to us while their symptoms are mild or moderate. Severe and chronic cases who have been wheelchair bound are too far gone, in my experience, to recover by any means.)

What in the world is going on? Why do so many people suffer with these symptoms?

I wouldn't have a clue except I'm a longtime student of what keeps people from being well and how we can help them. My first clue is my knowledge of the spine and how long term pressure on the spinal cord can cause a neuromuscular disorder and other bizarre syndromes. The second clue occurred after my friend and alternative medicine specialist Jacquelyn Chan D.O., recommended reading *Detoxify Or Die* by Sherry Rogers M.D.

Dr. Rogers discussed that neuromuscular disorders—those involving the nervous system and muscles—almost always have core causes of excess heavy metals and chemicals in the body. The brain 'short circuits' because of these toxins and can't control the muscles normally, thus the variety of tremors, weakness, and other muscle problems.

The key is to catch these cases early before they are too far advanced to help. I've been able to help a number of these with natural methods. Here's a testimonial from one of our success stories:

"My mobility had changed completely. I couldn't keep my balance while walking and fell down a lot with no warning. My speech changed for the worse and my handwriting was horrible. My hands and feet shook and I couldn't stop it. It seemed like something was wrong with the connection between my brain and muscles.

I was seen by many medical specialists in Columbus and at the Cleveland Clinic. They said I had MSA – Multiple System Atrophy. They don't know what causes it and there is no cure for it. It usually gets steadily worse with loss of movement, being bedridden, and then death.

Three years later, I was much worse and was losing hope. Then someone told me about advanced nutritional and chiropractic treatment that could help. After just a few months, I am almost totally normal! I haven't fallen down for months and my tremors are almost completely gone. Their treatment has given me my life back!"

In each of these ailments, we find excess chemicals and heavy metals affecting the brain. Sometimes, the nervous and immune systems have been stressed by—according to their medical specialists—antibiotics or flu shots. And we have to remove pressure from the spinal cord due to misaligned vertebrae.

Chemicals and heavy metals are everywhere—in the food, air, water, body care products, home furnishings, etc. . . . everywhere. Until big businesses put health concerns before profit, these toxins will abound. In the 1970s a popular phrase was: "Better living through chemistry." Forty years later, we're seeing the negative impacts on our health.

Some chemicals and heavy metals are purposely added to products, for example, aluminum in antiperspirant deodorants or mercury in vaccinations, dental fillings and processed foods. These are present in small amounts but, over time, can accumulate to excess amounts and contribute to physical and "mental" symptoms.

Certain individuals are *more sensitive* to these substances and are like a canary in a coalmine—a first line alert of coming danger to others.

The good news is that both chemicals and heavy metals can be minimized by lifestyle habits. And they can be removed with proper detox programs and taking personalized nutritional supplements that help the body remove these toxins. You definitely should get a personalized evaluation if you suffer with this condition. Until then, a good general program is listed below.

Don't wait until you or a loved one has received a diagnosis. Be proactive and regularly remove these toxins so you don't have to fight back from an illness. Make sure the bones of your spine are in alignment and not exerting slight but profound pressure on your spinal cord and nerves. As Benjamin Franklin noted many years ago, "An ounce of prevention is worth a pound of cure."

Medical *and* natural health care may both be needed for tough cases. Those doctors should communicate and work together so patients get well with the most effective and safe approaches.

Recommendations:

- ***21 Day Standard Process Purification Program to help remove chemicals and heavy metals:*** *Chlorella 6 and Cilantro 1 ½ droppers full (sip throughout the day after mixing in 16 ounces of water. Activate bottle in hot water for 30 minutes before using.)*
- ***supplements for muscles and nervous system:*** *Calcium Lactate 8, Magnesium Lactate 2, Cod Liver Oil 4, Tuna Omega Oil 4, Inositol 6, Cataplex B 6, Cataplex G 6*

Appendix S: Weight Loss

In my experience, the best way to reach and maintain your ideal weight is to regularly use healthy lifestyle habits: exercise, real food way of eating, whole food supplements, and holistic health care. My recommendations include:

1. *Wait until you are slightly hungry to eat again.*
1. *Avoid overeating.*
2. *When you start to feel hungry, drink a big glass of water. That will fill you up for a while before you really need a meal or snack.*
3. *Enjoy the real food way of eating and whole food supplements so you're not frequently snacking to find nutrients unavailable in junk and processed foods.*
4. *For the most part, avoid bedtime snacks except for a green drink, veggies, or bedtime tea.*
5. *Eat a wide variety of raw, sautéed, steamed, juiced, and powdered vegetables every day.*
6. *On your mirror and refrigerator, post pictures of how you want to look. Visualize yourself being trim and looking your very best.*
7. *Remember how important proper weight is for feeling great , reversing current health problems, and preventing future ones.*
8. *Weigh yourself weekly and measure monthly to monitor your progress and motivate yourself.*
9. *Have self pride! You have an amazing body; let it show!*
10. *Follow the Real Food Way of Eating as outlined in Diet chapter.*
11. *Regularly exercise as discussed in the Activity chapter.*
12. *Balance your endocrine system, liver, and pancreas with a nutrition-based healing approach.*

Metabolism is how your body makes and uses energy that is used for everything from cellular processes to exercising. Knowing how to efficiently metabolize calories translates into a leaner, healthier body.

A higher metabolism is a vital key to enjoying optimal weight. It contributes to having more energy, greater lean muscle, and less fat. This creates a positive cycle of being more active which, in turn, builds more muscle, burns more fat, and raises your metabolism even more.

Trim, energetic people have a race horse metabolism. They enjoy activity and can eat more food without gaining weight. Overweight people with lower activity levels, on the other hand, tend to have a slower or turtle metabolism. They have less energy and gain weight even though they may eat fewer calories.

Natural strategies for increasing your metabolic rate include:

1. ***Build lean body mass.*** *Your metabolic rate slows as you age, but increasing your amount of muscle counteracts the slowdown. More muscle mass increases the metabolic rate, burns calories more quickly, and burns body fat. Resistance training at least twice a week is essential for building more muscle and boosting your metabolism.*
2. ***Activity.*** *(see Activity chapter)*
3. ***Eat more!*** *Skipping meals or eating a low calorie diet makes your body think it's starving. To conserve energy, it lowers your metabolism. Eating three small meals with nutritious snacks in between if need signals that plenty of fuel is available so your body burn more calories.*
4. ***Minimize or avoid sugar.*** *As discussed, excess sugar intake is a sure road to gaining body fat and declining health.*
5. ***Drink tea.*** *Green and white tea stimulate metabolism longer than coffee and have other health benefits. This strategy is especially helpful for those who used to smoke cigarettes to lose weight.*
6. ***Drink more water.*** *Divide your body weight by two or three. That's how many ounces of water you should drink daily.*
7. ***Relax.*** *Extra stress increases cortisol, a hormone that decreases metabolism and increases weight gain especially at the waist.*
8. ***Eat real food.*** *You'll feel comfortably full after a moderately sized meal of fresh, healthy foods. Conversely, salt, sugar, and other chemicals in processed foods can make you overeat.*

9. ***Sleep more.*** *People who don't sleep at least seven to eight hours a night are more prone to weight gain. Also, lean muscle is regenerated in the last few hours of sleep.*

10. ***Eat sufficient protein.*** *Getting adequate protein each day helps build lean muscle mass, prevents hyperinsulinism, and aids fat burning. One rule of thumb for grams per day of protein is your body weight in pounds divided by 3.*

11. ***Get a nutritional health evaluation*** *to ensure that your thyroid and other metabolism related organs are functioning properly.*

12. ***Take whole food supplements*** *to provide genuine replacement parts so your body can be the lean self-monitoring and self-healing miracle it was designed to be. Taking supplements also prevents your body from wanting to graze for nutrients that aren't available in junk, processed, and overcooked foods. Recommendations include: Catalyn 6, Trace Minerals B12 (3), Cod Liver Oil 3, Calcium Lactate 6, ForTil B12 (3)*

Consistently follow these principles over time and you will likely lose pounds until you reach your ideal weight. The only exceptions might be those who suffer from significant genetic tendencies to overweight, and low metabolism due to irreversible health problems. In that case, definitely do #11.

References

Abrahamson, *E.M. Body, Mind, and Sugar*

Agatston, Arthur. *The South Beach Diet*

Anderson, Stephanie. *Why Your Doctor Offers Nutritional Supplements*

Ansley, Helen. *Life's Finishing School: Conscious Living, Conscious Dying*

Appleton, Nancy. *Lick the Sugar Habit*

Ballentine, Rudolph. *Diet and Nutrition: A Holistic Approach*

BhagavadGita

Bragg, Paul. *The Miracle of Fasting*

Braly, James and Holford, Patrick. *Hidden Food Allergies*

Brazelton, T. Barry. *Toddlers and Parents*

Buscaglia, Leo. *Living, Loving, and Learning*

Butterworth, Eric. *Discover the Power Within*

Butterworth, Eric. *Life Is For Loving*

Butterworth, Rev. Eric. *Life Is for Loving*

Campbell, Joseph. *An Open Life*

Campbell, Ryan. *Ready, Set, Go!*

Caplan, Theresa and Frank. *The Early Childhood Years*

Cheraskin and Ringsdorf. *Psychodietetics*

Collins, Susie and Otto. *Creating Relationship Trust*

Coulter, Harris and Fisher, Barbara. *A Shot in the Dark*

Cousins, Gabriel. *Spiritual Nutrition*

Cousins, Norman. *Anatomy of an Illness*

Dass, Ram and Gorman, Paul. *How Can I Help?*

Dass, Ram. Journey of Awakening: *A Meditator's Guidebook*

DeCava, Judith. *The Real Truth about Vitamins and AntiOxidants*

DeRoeck, Richard. *The Confusion About Chiropractors*

DouglasKlotz, Neil. *Prayers of the Cosmos*

Douglas, Ben. Ageless: *Living Younger Longer*

Dryburgh, Robert. *So You're Thinking of Going to a Chiropractor*

Dufty, William. *Sugar Blues*

Dyer, Wayne. *What Do You Really Want For Your Children?*

Dyer, Wayne. *You'll See It When You Believe It*

Eades, Michael and Mary. *The Protein Power Life Plan*

Ellis, Albert and Harper, Robert. *A Guide to Rational Living*

Errico, Rocco. *Let There Be Light*

Fallon, Sally and Enig, Mary. *Nourishing Traditions*

Forman, Robert. *How to Control Your Allergies*

Frankl, Victor. *Man's Search for Meaning*

Fredericks, Carlton. *PsychoNutrition*

Freeman and Dewolf. *Woulda, Coulda, Shoulda: Overcoming Regrets, Mistakes, and Missed Opportunities*

Fromm, Eric. *The Art of Loving*

Fuhrman, Joel. *Eat to Live*

Gerson, Max. *A Cancer Therapy—Results of 50 Cases*

Goleman, Daniel. *The Varieties of the Meditative Experience*

Green, Elmer and Green, Alyce. *Beyond Biofeedback*

Grinder and Bandler. *Reframing: NeuroLinguistic Programming and the Transformation of Meaning*

Hahn, Fredrick, Eades, Mary, and Eades, Michael. *The Slow Burn Fitness Revolution*

Hansel, Tim. *You Gotta Keep Dancin'*